Canadian Pharmacy Exams

Pharmacist OSCE Workbook

Dr. Fatima S. Marankan

Phi Publishing

Canadian Pharmacy Exams – Pharmacist OSCE Workbook

Copyright © 2019 by Phi Publishing

All rights reserved. No part of this publication may be reproduced, stored in a retrieval system, or transmitted in any form or by any means, electronic, mechanical, photocopying, recording, or otherwise, without the prior written permission of the copyrights owner.

Pharmacy is an ever-changing science. As new research and clinical experience broaden our knowledge, changes in treatment and drug therapy are needed. The author and contributors of Canadian Pharmacy Exams – Pharmacist OSCE Workbook have checked with resources believed to be reliable in their efforts to provide information that is complete and generally in accord with the standards accepted at the time of publication. However, in view of the possibility of human error or changes in medical sciences, neither the author nor any other party who has been involved in the preparation or publication of this work warrants that the information contained herein is in every respect accurate or complete and they disclaim all responsibility for any errors or omissions or for the results obtained from the use of the information contained in this work.

Library and Archives Canada Cataloguing in Publication

Phi Publishing
Canadian Pharmacy Exams Pharmacist OSCE Workbook / Author, Dr. Fatima S. Marankan – 3rd Canadian Edition.

About the Author

Dr. Marankan holds a postgraduate degree in pharmacy from the College of Pharmacy at UIC, USA coupled with extensive experience in pharmacy instruction at the University of British Columbia, Canada. Dr. Marankan was recently a visiting medical professor. Her academic, research and teaching achievements have been recognized by the Paul Sang Award at the University of Illinois at Chicago and the TLEF Award at the University of British Columbia, Canada. Furthermore, Dr. Marankan was the lead consultant in the development and implementation of OSCE training in Vancouver, Canada.

Throughout her education and career as pharmacy instructor at the University of British Columbia, Fatima has gained extensive understanding of the requirements of pharmacy licensing exams in Canada. This knowledge has guided the development of the Canadian Pharmacy Exams Series:

- Pharmacist Evaluating Exam Practice - Volume 1
- Pharmacist Evaluating Exam Practice – Volume 2
- Pharmacist MCQ Review
- Pharmacist OSCE Workbook
- Pharmacy Technician MCQ Review
- Pharmacy Technician OSPE Workbook

Thank you to all contributing reviewers!

Preface

The Qualifying Exam Part II or Objective Structured Clinical Examination (OSCE) is a primary exam towards Canadian pharmacy licensure. The OSCE has been designed to evaluate the knowledge and practical skills of Canadian Pharmacy Graduates and International Pharmacy Graduates seeking licensure. A candidate for the OSCE must be prepared to demonstrate practical skills in simulated-stations by interacting with a Standardized Patient (SP), Standardized Client (SC) or Standardized Health Professional (SHP). Stations are designed to evaluate several skills such as:

- Interviewing and collecting relevant patient information
- Interpretation of patient information to identify potential drug-drug interactions
- Interpretation of patient information to identify and manage drug adverse reactions
- Interpretation of patient information to identify the need for alternate drug therapy regimen
- Assess patient's health status and address concerns
- Collaborating with other healthcare professionals to meet patient needs
- Ability to address ethical issues
- Effective and trusting communication with a patient

The Qualifying Exam Part I (MCQ) and The Qualifying Exam Part II (OSCE) address the following nine competencies as per the Pharmacy Examining Board of Canada (PEBC®):

- Patient Care
- Health Promotion
- Intra and Inter-Professional Collaboration
- Knowledge and Research Application
- Ethical, Legal and Professional Responsibilities
- Quality and Safety
- Communication and Education
- Product Distribution
- Practice Setting

Canadian Pharmacy Exams™ - Pharmacist OSCE Workbook is designed as a self-study or group-study tool to help the student seeking pharmacy licensure in Canada test his/her exam readiness, identify areas of strength and weakness. The book provides an extensive opportunity to test and improve relevant practical skills within the nine competencies listed above. The workbook contains 55 Interactive Cases/Stations, 47 Non-Interactive Cases/Stations, blank forms to solve cases, an assessment form and an OSCE Checklist. *NEW STATIONS!!*

All cases are supplemented by detailed solutions and explanations to ensure further understanding and learning of new concepts. These comments are truly the keystone of Canadian Pharmacy Exams™. We trust that each Canadian Pharmacy Exams™ book is a valuable learning and self-assessment tool towards Canadian Pharmacy licensure. The following book is now available at Amazon:
Canadian Pharmacy Exams™ - Pharmacist MCQ Review

Trusted Convenient Comprehensive Canadian Pharmacy Exams™ Online Review for Pharmacists and Pharmacy Technicians at www.cpepreponline.com

FREE Computer-Based Exam Readiness Tests
FREE Pharmacy Resources

References

- Compendium of Therapeutic Choices, 2019
- Compendium of Pharmaceuticals and Specialties, 2019
- Compendium of Products for Minor Ailments, 2019
- Rx Files, 2017
- Drug Facts and Comparisons, 2017

Content

HOW TO USE OSCE WORKBOOK	07
OSCE CHECKLIST	09
OSCE ASSESSMENT FORM	10
INTERACTIVE CASES	12
NON-INTERACTIVE CASES	260

HOW TO USE OSCE WORKBOOK

Interactive Cases/Stations

55 Interactive Cases *3 New Stations!!*

First, review the OSCE Checklist. The checklist is the roadmap that helps you navigate step-by-step the process of solving, effectively, each interactive station. It highlights important points to be addressed during your interaction with a Standardized Patient (SP)

Self-Study Option

You have 7 minutes to complete each station. Time yourself!

1. Make sure to have access to suggested references for the station.
2. As a replacement for Candidate Notebook, a Case Review Form is included to each station. Use the form to write useful notes as you review the station. For self-study, you may use the same Case Review Form to show how you would solve the case. If applicable, fill the Candidate Answer Sheet/Prescription Review Sheet.
3. Review the Solution following the completion of the station. Compare the Solution to your Case Review Form to evaluate your performance.

Practice, Practice, Practice …

Group-Study Option

A group of three candidates is suggested.

You have 7 minutes to complete each station.

1. Assign each candidate to one of the following three roles:

- OSCE Candidate. Have a copy of Candidate Instructions and Questions including Patient Profile, if available, Case Review Form (Candidate Notebook) and Candidate Answer Sheet/Prescription Review Sheet if applicable. Have access to suggested references for the station.
- Standardized Patient (SP), Standardized Client (SC) or Standardized Health Professional (SHP) depending on the station. Have a copy of SP, SC or SHP Instructions including Patient Profile if available.
- OSCE Assessor. Have a copy of the Assessment Form and Solution. Time the candidate!

2. Review and discuss the Solution following the completion of the station.

Practice, Practice, Practice …

Important Tip: Make sure to use role reversal by playing the patient at least twice. Role reversal is a powerful technique proven to enhance the counselling skills of healthcare professionals. It improves significantly your understanding of patient expectations and concerns.

Non-interactive Cases/Stations

47 Non-Interactive Cases divided in two sections: Prescription Labels Stations and New Prescriptions Stations. Each station has 3, 4 or 5 prescriptions.
You have 7 minutes to complete each station. Time yourself!
Make sure you have a recent copy of Compendium of Pharmaceuticals and Specialties (CPS) for New Prescription Cases.
Review the Answer Key following the completion of the station. Evaluate for performance.

OSCE Checklist

1. Introduce yourself and identify the patient

2. Collect patient information
   Have you taken the medication before?
   If yes, ask about effectiveness, adverse reactions and concerns
   If no, ask about what the doctor told the patient about the medication (new Rx)
   Ask about other drugs use (Rx and OTCs)
   Ask about allergies

3. Educate the patient about the drug
   Drug name
   Why the drug is used?
   How it works?
   How to use?
   How long to use?
   Proper storage
   If appropriate, provide refill information
   Any applicable instructions such as inhaler, nasal spray, eye drops, patch….

4. Discuss major adverse effects
   What to expect?
   How to manage adverse effects if applicable?
   Will adverse effects go away with time or not?
   What to do if intolerable?

5. Discuss major drug related interactions
   Drug-drug (Rx and OTCs)
   Drug-food/nutrients
   Drug-herbal products

6. If applicable, discuss self-monitoring such as blood pressure, blood sugar, body temperature ….
   Explain the purpose of monitoring
   Explain how to use monitoring device

7. Summarize and assess patient understanding (e.g. Could you tell me how you should use this medication? Could you show me how to use the inhaler? Do you have any questions?.....) *Note: Customize depending on time remaining*
   Encourage the patient to contact the pharmacy with any questions.

OSCE ASSESSMENT FORM

Communication skills (circle one)

4. Appropriate
3. Appropriate/Marginal
2. Poor/Marginal
1. Poor

Comments

Outcome (circle one)

4. Problem solved
3. Problem marginally solved
2. Problem not solved
1. Problem not identified

Comments

Performance (circle one)

4. Meets expectations
3. Meets expectations marginally
2. Does not meet expectations
1. Unacceptable

Comments

Information inaccuracy   Yes   No

Risk to patient's safety   Yes   No

Overall Mark

PASS   FAIL

Interactive Case #1: Entocort Enema for Ulcerative Colitis
Pharmacist – Standardized Patient Interaction

Your (Candidate) instructions

Case description:

A male patient who has been recently diagnosed with ulcerative colitis comes to see you with a new prescription for Entocort Enema. He has some questions and concerns regarding the use of the medication. It is his first prescription for Entocort Enema. He is confident the pharmacist will help. Assist the patient as you would in practice.

This station must be completed in 7 minutes

Station materials and references:
Patient profile
Compendium of Pharmaceuticals and Specialties (CPS)
Entocort Enema

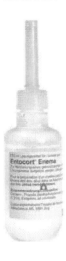

Patient profile

Patient Name: James Kim
Gender: Male
Age: 38 years old
Allergies: None known
Medical History: Ulcerative Colitis (just diagnosed)
Current medications (Rx & nRx): Daily Centrum Multivitamin, Tylenol prn for occasional headaches
New prescription: Entocort Enema daily for 4 weeks
Social/lifestyle: Elementary school teacher, non-smoker, moderate alcohol intake – 3 to 5 drinks weekly, runs at least 4 times weekly

Standardized patient introductions and questions

<u>Case description</u>:

A male patient who has been recently diagnosed with ulcerative colitis comes to see the pharmacist with a new prescription for Entocort Enema. He has some questions and concerns regarding the use of the medication. It is his first prescription for Entocort Enema. He is confident the pharmacist will help.

Patient profile

Patient Name: James Kim
Gender: Male
Age: 38 years old
Allergies: None known
Medical History: Ulcerative Colitis (just diagnosed)
Current medications (Rx & nRx): Daily Centrum Multivitamin, Tylenol prn for occasional headaches
New prescription: Entocort Enema daily for 4 weeks

"Hi, I just got this new prescription from my doctor. I am not sure how to use. Could you also tell me what to expect?"
If not addressed by the candidate after 4 minutes, the standardized patient will ask the following questions:
What should I expect while on this medication?
How should I use it?
For how long should I use it?
When would be the best time to use it?

CASE REVIEW FORM
Write notes, answers, interview and counselling to show how you would solve this case

Solution - Interactive Case #1

<u>Primary goals</u>:

- Discuss why the drug is being used
- Discuss how the drug works
- Discuss common adverse reactions
- Explain how to use Entocort Enema

The candidate is expected to discuss:

- Entocort Enema is used to treat ulcerative colitis localized in the rectum and the lower large bowel. Ulcerative colitis is caused by inflammation in the bowel wall.
- Entocort (budesonide) belongs to the class of glucocorticosteroids that are used to reduce inflammation. The medication is placed directly in the rectum to reduce inflammation.
- The most common adverse reactions are flatulence, nausea, diarrhea, skin rash and/or itching.
- One Entocort (budesonide) Enema should be administered daily in the evening before going to bed for 4 weeks.
- Entocort Enema is reconstituted by adding one dispersible tablet into the enema bottle, then the bottle is vigorously shaken for at least 10 seconds or until the tablet is completely dissolved. The tablet will dissolve rapidly and the suspension will turn slightly yellowish.
- Each carton contains 7 dispersible tablets and vehicle solutions. Store at 15-30°C. After preparation of the enema, the solution is intended for immediate use.

How to prepare and use Entocort Enema
- 1. Remove the nozzle, with the protective cap on, from the bottle.
- 2. Take a tablet from the aluminum foil pack and put it into the bottle.
- 3. Put the nozzle back on the bottle and make sure that the protective cap is firmly on. Shake the bottle vigorously for at least 10 seconds or until the tablet has dissolved and a slightly yellowish liquid has been formed. A plastic bag has been enclosed which you may use to protect your hand when you administer the enema.
- 4. Lie down on your left side. Shake the bottle again before removing the protective cap. Empty the contents into the rectum. Then, remove the plastic bag from your hand by pulling it over the bottle
- 5. Roll over on your stomach. Stay in this position for 5 minutes.
- 6. Choose a suitable position to sleep in. Try to retain the enema as long as possible, preferably for the whole night.
- Maintain a well-balanced diet with supplements
- Summarize and confirm that patient understands

Interactive Case #2: Adalat XL Plus for Hypertension
Pharmacist – Standardized Patient Interaction

Your (Candidate) instructions

Case description:

A male patient who has been on Adalat XL for the treatment of hypertension comes to see you with a new prescription for Adalat XL Plus. Assist the patient as you would in practice.

This station must be completed in 7 minutes

Station materials and references:

Patient profile
Compendium of Pharmaceuticals and Specialties (CPS)

Patient profile

Patient Name: John Williams
Gender: Male
Age: 56 years old
Allergies: None known
Medical History: Hypertension diagnosed 5 months ago
Current medications (Rx & nRx): Adalat XL (last filled one month ago), daily aspirin 81 mg, daily Centrum Multivitamin
New prescription: Adalat XL Plus 30 mg qd x 3 months
Social/lifestyle: Writer, non-smoker, no alcohol intake

Standardized patient introductions and questions

<u>Case description</u>:

A male patient who has been on Adalat XL for the treatment of hypertension comes to see the pharmacist with a new prescription for Adalat XL Plus.

Patient profile

Patient Name: John Williams
Gender: Male
Age: 56 years old
Allergies: None known
Medical History: Hypertension diagnosed 5 months ago
Current medications (Rx & nRx): Adalat XL (last filled one month ago), daily aspirin 81 mg, daily Centrum Multivitamin
New prescription: Adalat XL Plus 30 mg qd x 3 months
Social/lifestyle: Writer, non-smoker, no alcohol intake

"Hi, I just got this new prescription from my doctor. I have been using a similar product for few months. Do I need to take the new medication and the old one? Is there anything I need to know about the new product?"

If not addressed by the candidate after 4 minutes, the standardized patient will ask the following questions:

Should I take the new medication with my old one?
How should I use this new product?
Should I keep using my baby aspirin?
The package has pink pills and blue pills. Could you tell me which one is aspirin?
What should I do if I forget my pills?

CASE REVIEW FORM
Write notes, answers, interview and counselling to show how you would solve this case

Solution – Interactive Case #2

<u>Primary goals:</u>

- Ask about his experience using Adalat XL (effectiveness, side effects, concerns….)
- Explain that his previous medication Adalat XL is being replaced with Adalat XL Plus
- Explain that Adalat XL Plus contains both Adalat XL and Aspirin 81 mg. Therefore, there is no need to take aspirin 81 mg separately (refer to profile)
- Explain how to take Adalat XL Plus including missed dose management
- Recall common adverse reactions and dietary warning (grapefruit juice)

The candidate is expected to discuss:

Adalat XL Plus contains both Adalat XL and Aspirin 81 mg. Therefore, there is no need to take aspirin 81 mg separately; antihypertensive agent and platelet aggregation inhibitor
ADALAT XL PLUS is a Convenience Pack containing Adalat XL 30 mg XL packed with Aspirin 81 mg tablets. The tablets are packaged in clear blisters and are arranged side by side. Adalat XL tablets are round and dusty rose and Aspirin 81 mg tablets are pale blue.
Take 1 tablet of Adalat XL (nifedipine extended-release tablet) and 1 tablet of Aspirin 81 mg (acetylsalicylic acid enteric coated tablet) daily preferably after meals with plenty of water. Adalat XL and aspirin tablets must be swallowed whole and should not be bitten or divided. Take the tablets ideally at the same time every day. The medication is slowly released over 18 hours.
DO NOT eat grapefruit or drink grapefruit juice while you are using this medication.
The most common adverse effects of Adalat XL are edema, headache, fatigue, dizziness, constipation, and nausea. The most common side effect of aspiring are: stomach pain, heartburn, and nausea
Adalat XL Plus should be stored at room temperature (15-30°C). Protect from light and humidity.
If applicable, encourage the patient to return unused Adalat XL pills to the pharmacy.

Missed Dose Management
If you miss a pill, use it as soon as you can. If it is almost time for your next pill, wait until then to use the medication and skip the missed dose. Do not take extra medication to make up for a missed pill.
Recall non-pharmacology strategies for the management of hypertension such as physical activity (*physical activity is lacking in his profile*), DASH diet and stress management
Summarize and confirm that patient understands

Interactive Case #3: Androgel 1%
Pharmacist – Standardized Patient Interaction

Your (Candidate) Instructions

Case description:

Mr. Ryan is one of your regular patients. He is visiting your pharmacy to fill a new prescription for Androgel 1% for the treatment of erectile dysfunction and reduced libido associated with low testosterone. He has some questions and concerns regarding the use of the medication. It is his first prescription for Androgel. Assist the patient as you would in practice.

This station must be completed in 7 minutes

Station materials and references:

Patient profile
Compendium of Pharmaceuticals and Specialties (CPS)

Patient profile

Patient Name: Robert Ryan
Gender: Male
Age: 52 years old
Allergies: None known
Medical History: Hyperlipidemia
Current medications (Rx & nRx): Crestor 40 mg qd, Omega 3 supplements, Tylenol prn for occasional headaches, daily Multivitamin
New prescription: Androgel 1% pump, 50 mg testosterone daily
Social/lifestyle: Accountant, non-smoker, moderate alcohol intake – 3 to 5 drinks weekly, daily physical activity.

Standardized patient introductions and questions

<u>Case description</u>:

Mr. Ryan is a regular patient at the pharmacy. He is visiting the pharmacy to fill a new prescription for Androgel 1% for the treatment of erectile dysfunction and reduced libido associated with low testosterone. He has some questions and concerns regarding the use of the medication. It is his first prescription for Androgel.

Patient profile

Patient Name: Robert Ryan
Gender: Male
Age: 52 years old
Allergies: None known
Medical History: Hyperlipidemia
Current medications (Rx & nRx): Crestor 40 mg qd, Omega 3 supplements, Tylenol prn for occasional headaches, daily Multivitamin
New prescription: Androgel 1% pump, 50 mg testosterone daily
Social/lifestyle: Accountant, non-smoker, moderate alcohol intake – 3 to 5 drinks weekly, daily physical activity

"Hi, I just got this new prescription from my doctor. I am not sure how to use. Could you also tell me what to expect?"
If not addressed by the candidate after 4 minutes, the standardized patient will ask the following questions:
Where should I apply it?
What is the amount of gel needed?
How long should I leave it on before taking a shower?
What should I expect while on this medication?

CASE REVIEW FORM
Write notes, answers, interview and counselling to show how you would solve this case

Solution – Interactive Case #3

<u>Primary goals</u>:

- Discuss why the drug is being used
- Discuss how the drug works
- Explain how to use Androgel
- Discuss common adverse reactions
- Discuss warnings and precautions

The candidate is expected to discuss:
Androgel is indicated for testosterone replacement therapy in adult males for conditions associated with a deficiency or absence of endogenous testosterone (hypogonadism).
Androgel is a clear, colorless, fragrance free, hydroalcoholic gel containing 1% testosterone.
Androgel provides continuous transdermal delivery of testosterone for 24 hours following a single application to intact, clean, dry skin of the shoulders, upper arms and/or abdomen.
The most adverse effects are: acne, prostate disorder (increased prostate specific antigen), irritation of application site, increased red blood cells, and increased cholesterol. *Recommend cholesterol monitoring due to history of hyperlipidemia* (refer to profile).

Apply 5 g of 1% gel (provide 50 mg testosterone) once daily, preferably in the morning, to clean, dry, intact skin of the shoulders and upper arms and/or abdomen.
The metered-dose pump contains 60 actuations. The pump delivers 1.25 g of gel for each actuation. 4 actuations provide the required daily dose of 5 g or 50 mg testosterone.
Application sites should be allowed to dry for a few minutes prior to dressing.
Hands should be washed with soap and water immediately after Androgel has been applied.

Notes on Administration
- Androgel should not be applied to the scrotum.
- Androgel should be applied daily to clean, dry, healthy, intact skin.
- For optimal absorption of testosterone, wait at least 5-6 hours after application prior to showering or swimming. Showering or swimming after just 1 hour should have a minimal effect on absorption.

Serious Warnings and Precautions
Virilization has been reported in children and adult women who were secondarily exposed to Androgel. Advise patients to strictly adhere to the following recommended instructions for use to minimize the potential for secondary exposure to Androgel.
- Children and women should avoid contact with unwashed or unclothed application site(s) of men using testosterone gel.
- Androgel should only be applied to the shoulders, upper arms, and/ or abdomen. The area of application should be limited to the area that will be covered by a short sleeve t-shirt.

When a shirt is used to cover the application site(s), the transfer of Androgel from the male to the female partner can be completely prevented.
- Patients should wash their hands immediately with soap and water after applying Androgel.
- Patients should cover the application site(s) with clothing (e.g., a shirt) after the gel has dried.
- Prior to any situation in which skin-to-skin contact with the application site is anticipated, patients should wash the application site(s) thoroughly with soap and water to remove any testosterone residue.
- In the events that unwashed or unclothed skin to which Androgel has been applied and/or that the testosterone gel user's unwashed shirts and/ or other fabrics (such as towels and sheets) come in direct contact with the skin of another person, the general area of contact on the other person should be washed with soap and water as soon as possible. Residual testosterone is removed from the skin surface by washing with soap and water.
- Gels are flammable. Following application of Androgel, allow gel to dry completely before smoking or going near an open flame.

Summarize and confirm that patient understands

Interactive Case #4: Treatment of conjunctivitis
Pharmacist – Standardized Patient Interaction

Your (Candidate) Instructions

Case description:

A young female patient who has been recently diagnosed with bacterial conjunctivitis comes to see you with a new prescription for Zaditor. She has some questions and concerns regarding the use of the medication. Assist the patient as you would in practice.

This station must be completed in 7 minutes

Station materials and references:

Patient profile
Compendium of Pharmaceuticals and Specialties (CPS)
Compendium of Therapeutic Choices (CTC)

Patient profile

Patient Name: Anita Chan
Gender: Female
Age: 23 years old
Allergies: None known
Medical History: None
Current medications (Rx & nRx): Daily Multivitamin
New prescription: Zaditor 2.5 mg, 1 drop in both eyes q12h
Social/lifestyle: Student, non-smoker, 2 to 3 alcoholic drinks weekly, yoga 5 times weekly

Standardized patient introductions and questions

<u>Case description</u>:

A young female patient who has been recently diagnosed with bacterial conjunctivitis comes to see the pharmacist with a new prescription for Zaditor. She has some questions and concerns regarding the use of the medication.

Patient profile

Patient Name: Anita Chan
Gender: Female
Age: 23 years old
Allergies: None known
Medical History: None
Current medications (Rx & nRx): Daily Multivitamin
New prescription: Zaditor 2.5 mg, 1 drop in both eyes q12h
Social/lifestyle: Student, non-smoker, 2 to 3 alcoholic drinks weekly, yoga 5 times weekly

"Hi, I just got this new prescription from my doctor. I am not sure how to use. Could you also tell me what to expect?"
If not addressed by the candidate after 4 minutes, the standardized patient will ask the following questions:
How long it takes to work?
How many drops do I need?
How often should I use it?

CASE REVIEW FORM

Write notes, answers, interview and counselling to show how you would solve this case

Solution – Interactive Case #4

Primary goals:

- Determine that Zaditor is used for the treatment of allergic conjunctivitis not bacterial conjunctivitis
- Call the physician to identify an appropriate course of action

The candidate is expected to discuss:
Zaditor is use for the treatment of allergic conjunctivitis not bacterial conjunctivitis.
Reassure the patient. Call her physician to identify an appropriate course of action.
Summarize and confirm that patient understands

Overview of Zaditor
Zaditor (Ketotifen) is a fast acting non-competitive histamine antagonist (H1-receptor). In addition, ketotifen inhibits the release of mediators from mast cells involved in hypersensitivity reactions. Zaditor prevents ocular itching and redness associated with allergic conjunctivitis within minutes after administration and last up to 12 hours.

Interactive Case #5: Terazol 3 Dual-Pak
Pharmacist – Standardized Patient Interaction

Your (Candidate) instructions

Case description:

A female patient who has been recently diagnosed with vaginal yeast infection comes to see you with a new prescription for Terazol 3 Dual-Pak. She has some questions and concerns regarding the use of the medication. Assist the patient as you would in practice.

This station must be completed in 7 minutes

Station materials and references:

Patient profile
Compendium of Pharmaceuticals and Specialties (CPS)

Patient profile

Patient Name: Mary William
Gender: Female
Age: 28 years old
Allergies: None known
Medical History: Vaginal yeast infection (just diagnosed)
Current medications (Rx & nRx): Daily Centrum Multivitamin, Tylenol prn for occasional headaches, Omega 3 supplements
New prescription: Terazol 3 Dual-Pak
Social/lifestyle: Dance instructor, non-smoker, moderate alcohol intake – 3 to 5 drinks weekly

Standardized patient introductions and questions

Case description:

A female patient who has been recently diagnosed with vaginal yeast infection comes to see you with a new prescription for Terazol 3 Dual-Pak. She has some questions and concerns regarding the use of the medication.

Patient profile

Patient Name: Mary William
Gender: Female
Age: 28 years old
Allergies: None known
Medical History: Vaginal yeast infection (just diagnosed)
Current medications (Rx & nRx): Daily Centrum Multivitamin, Tylenol prn for occasional headaches, Omega 3 supplements
New prescription: Terazol 3 Dual-Pak
Social/lifestyle: Dance instructor, non-smoker, moderate alcohol intake – 3 to 5 drinks weekly

Start by saying: "Hi, I just got this new prescription from my doctor. I am not sure how to use. Could you also tell me what to expect?"
If not addressed by the candidate after 4 minutes, the standardized patient must ask the following questions:
How should I use it?
For how long should I use it?
Do I swallow the pills?
When would be the best time to use it?

CASE REVIEW FORM

Write notes, answers, interview and counselling to show how you would solve this case

Solution - Interactive Case #5

Primary goals:

- Discuss why the drug is being used
- Discuss how the drug works
- Explain how to use the medication
- Discuss common adverse reactions

The candidate is expected to discuss:

This medication is an azole antifungal. It works by stopping the growth of yeast (fungus) that causes the infection.
Terazol (terconazole) 3 Dual-Pak contains three 80 mg ovules, a vaginal applicator and 9 g tube of terconazole 0.8% vaginal cream.

Administration instructions
One Terazol Vaginal Ovule (80 mg of terconazole) is administered intravaginally once daily at bedtime for three consecutive days. In addition, a thin layer of Terazol Vaginal Cream (0.8% terconazole) is applied for three consecutive days directly to the vulva and massaged in gently.
Common adverse effects are: headache, genital burning, dysmenorrhea (painful menstruation), genital pruritus, genital pain and discomfort
Advise the patient not to use vaginal contraceptive diaphragms or condoms with Terazol ovules. The formulation base used in the ovule formulation may interact with certain natural rubber products, such as those used in vaginal contraceptive diaphragms or condoms.
Terazol cream and ovules should be discontinued and patients should not be re-treated if sensitization, vulvovaginal irritation, fever, chills or flu-like symptoms are experienced during treatment. Advise the patient to contact her physician if she has any of the symptoms.
Non pharmacologic preventive strategies: drink milk or eat yogurt containing lactobacillus, wear cotton or cotton-lined under wear, avoid feminine sprays, perfumes and douche, wipe vaginal area from front to back.
Summarize and confirm that patient understands

Interactive Case #6: Endometriosis
Pharmacist – Standardized Patient Interaction

Your (Candidate) instructions

Case description:

A female patient is visiting your pharmacy with a new prescription for Synarel. Mrs. Singh has been recently diagnosed with endometriosis. She has some questions and concerns regarding the use of the medication and potential adverse effects. Assist the patient as you would in practice.

This station must be completed in 7 minutes

Station materials and references:

Patient profile
Compendium of Pharmaceuticals and Specialties (CPS)

Patient profile

Patient Name: Karen Singh
Gender: Female
Age: 48 years old
Allergies: Aspirin
Medical History: Urinary Tract Infection, Endometriosis (just diagnosed)
Current medications (Rx & nRx): Daily Centrum Multivitamin, Drixoral Nasal Decongestant, Tylenol prn for back pain, Omega 3 supplements, Probiotic supplements
New prescription: Synarel 2mg/ml, 400 ug daily for 6 months
Social/lifestyle: Stay Home Mom, non-smoker, no alcohol intake, daily walk

Standardized patient introductions and questions

Case description:

A female patient is visiting the pharmacy with a new prescription for Synarel. Mrs. Singh has been recently diagnosed with endometriosis. She has some questions and concerns regarding the use of the medication and potential adverse effects.

Patient profile

Patient Name: Karen Singh
Gender: Female
Age: 48 years old
Allergies: Aspirin
Medical History: Urinary Tract Infection, Endometriosis (just diagnosed)
Current medications (Rx & nRx): Daily Centrum Multivitamin, Drixoral Nasal Decongestant, Tylenol prn for back pain, Omega 3 supplements, Probiotic supplements
New prescription: Synarel 2mg/ml, 400 ug daily for 6 months
Social/lifestyle: Stay Home Mom, non-smoker, no alcohol intake, daily walk

"Hi, I just got this new prescription from my doctor. I am not sure how to use. Could you also tell me what to expect?"
If not addressed by the candidate after 4 minutes, the standardized patient must ask the following questions:
How should I use it?
How many sprays do I need?
For how long should I use it?
How about my other nasal spray?
Can I use the two medications (nasal sprays) together?

CASE REVIEW FORM
Write notes, answers, interview and counselling to show how you would solve this case

Solution - Interactive Case #6

<u>Primary goals</u>:

- Discuss why the drug is being used
- Discuss how the drug works
- Explain how to use the medication
- Discuss common adverse reactions

The candidate is expected to discuss:

Synarel (nafarelin) is indicated for hormonal management of endometriosis, including pain relief and reduction of endometriotic lesions.

Nafarelin is an agonistic analogue of the gonadotropin releasing hormone (GnRH). Given as a single intranasal dose, nafarelin stimulates release of the pituitary gonadotropins, LH and FSH, with consequent increase of ovarian steroidogenesis (production of steroids). Repeated intranasal dosing abolishes the stimulatory effect on the pituitary gland.

Twice daily administration of 200 µg, as a nasal spray, leads to decreased secretion of gonadal steroids by about 4 weeks resulting in the regression and atrophy of endometrium tissue.

Make a note on a calendar on the day starting a new bottle of Synarel Nasal Spray. Keep track of each dose.

The most frequently reported adverse events associated with hypoestrogenic effects are: hot flashes, decrease in libido, headache, vaginal dryness, mood disturbances, acne, myalgia and reduction in breast size. Nasal irritation is also likely.

Administration instructions
- One spray (200 µg of nafarelin) into one nostril in the morning and one spray into the other nostril in the evening for 6 months
- Treatment should be started between days 2 and 4 of the menstrual cycle.
- Each bottle contains 8 ml of Synarel and provides a 30 day supply (about 60 sprays).

Priming

Before you use a bottle of Synarel Nasal Spray for the first time you have to prime the spray pump by following these steps:

1. Remove the safety clip and the clear plastic dust cover from the spray bottle.
2. Put two fingers on the "shoulders" of the spray bottle and put your thumb on the bottom of the bottle.
3. Hold the bottle in an upright position away from you. Apply pressure EVENLY to the "shoulders" and push down QUICKLY AND FIRMLY until a fine spray occurs. Usually the spray will appear after about 5 to 10 pumps.
4. The pump is now primed. Priming only needs to be done once when you start using a new bottle of Synarel Nasal Spray.

Using the spray
1. Gently blow your nose to clear both nostrils before you use Synarel Nasal Spray.
2. Remove the safety clip and clear plastic dust cover from the spray bottle.
3. Clean the tip of pump with a clean soft cloth.
4. Bend your head slightly forward and put the spray tip into one nostril.
5. Close the other nostril with your finger.
6. Applying pressure EVENLY to the "shoulders", QUICKLY AND FIRMLY pump the sprayer ONE TIME, at the same time as you sniff in gently.
7. Remove the sprayer from your nose and tilt your head backwards for a few seconds. This lets the spray spread over the back of your nose.
9. Clean the tip of the pump.
10. Replace the safety clip and the clear plastic dust cover on the spray bottle.

Missed dose management

It is very important that you do not miss a single dose of Synarel. However, if you do miss a dose, follow the directions below.

If it is almost time for your next dose, skip the dose you missed and take your next dose when you are meant to. Otherwise, take it as soon as you remember and then go back to taking it as you would normally. Do not take a double dose to make up for the dose that you missed.

If you miss one or more doses, vaginal bleeding (breakthrough bleeding) may occur.

Make a note on a calendar on the day starting a new bottle of Synarel Nasal Spray. Keep track of each dose.

Advise the patient not to use her nasal decongestant (refer to profile) until at least 30 minutes after Synarel is applied.

Summarize and confirm that patient understands

Interactive case #7: Ethic
Pharmacist – Standardized Client Interaction

Your (Candidate) instructions

Case description:

You are working in the hospital pharmacy. Karyn and her husband, George, are visiting to fill a new prescription for fentanyl for the management of cancer pain. Her husband is leaving the hospital following surgery. Unfortunately, his liver cancer is inoperable; the surgeons were not able to remove the tumor. Mr. Dean is terminally ill. Karyn gave you the prescription and whispered not to tell her husband George about his condition. Assist the client as you would in practice.

This station must be completed in 7 minutes

Station materials and references:

None

Standardized client introductions and questions

Case description:

Karyn and her husband, George, are visiting the hospital pharmacy to fill a new prescription for fentanyl for the management of cancer pain. Her husband is leaving the hospital following surgery. Unfortunately, his liver cancer is inoperable; the surgeons were not able to remove the tumor. Mr. Dean is terminally ill. Karyn gave the prescription to the pharmacist and whispered not to tell her husband George about his condition.
Karyn continues to address you:
"He needs his strength now to recover from the surgery. If you tell him he's going to be so upset it will make him worse."
"We have been married for almost 45 years. I know my husband's personality. He has also recently lost a friend to lung cancer. I just want the best for him."
"Are you going to tell him? Isn't it your duty to prolong his life? Why do you have to tell him?"
"It's easy for you; you probably won't see him again. I'm going to have to live with him and watch how destroyed he will be."

CASE REVIEW FORM
Write notes, answers, interview and counselling to show how you would solve this case

Solution - Interactive case #7

Candidate is expected to:

Investigate further why she does not want him to know about his condition.
Explain that he will probably ask about the diagnosis and he may lose trust in family and healthcare professionals
Explain that it could be beneficial for the patient to know and put affairs in order or do things knowing he has a limited time left.
Explain that a healthcare professional cannot lie to a patient. Principle of veracity.
State that the patient has the right to know.
Explain that if asked directly, you have to tell the truth. However if not asked, you will not tell more than what the patient desires to know.
Refuse to promise not to tell.

Interactive case #8: Ethic
Pharmacist – Standardized Client Interaction

Your (Candidate) instructions

Case description:

An undercover police detective, Mr. Cameron is in the pharmacy to talk to you. One of the pharmacy regular patients, Mr. Paul Ryan, has been on the police watch list for about three months. Mr. Ryan is suspected to be involved in several gang criminal activities. Despite the detectives consistent efforts they have not been able to confirm his residence. Fortunately, Detective Cameron who has been following Mr. Paul Ryan today spotted him leaving your pharmacy. Detective Cameron is requesting access the Paul's profile to finally confirm his residence. Please, assist Detective Cameron as you would in practice.

This station must be completed in 7 minutes

Station materials and references:

None

Standardized client introductions and questions

Case description:

An undercover police detective, Mr. Cameron is in the pharmacy to talk to the pharmacist on duty. One of the pharmacy regular patients, Mr. Paul Ryan, has been on the police watch list for about three months. Mr. Ryan is suspected to be involved in several gang criminal activities. Despite the detectives consistent efforts they have not been able to confirm his residence. Fortunately, Detective Cameron who has been following Mr. Paul Ryan today spotted him leaving the pharmacy. Detective Cameron is requesting access the Paul's profile to finally confirm his residence.

"Hi, I am Detective John Cameron (*shows ID*). We have been watching closely, Paul Ryan, who just left your pharmacy. He is suspected to be involved in several criminal activities in the community. I just need quick access to his file to confirm his residence. It won't take long."
During his interaction with the pharmacist, Detective Cameron continues by saying:
"I am not interested in his medical information; I just need to check his address. Is that too much to ask?"
"We need to solve this case fast! We don't have much time to waste."
"Can't you make an exception?"

CASE REVIEW FORM
Write notes, answers, interview and counselling to show how you would solve this case

Solution - Interactive case #8

The candidate is expected to:

Explain that patient's information is confidential.
Explain that confidentiality is not limited to medical condition and medication use; all information (including residence) collected from the patient is viewed as confidential and must be treated as such.
Reassure the Detective that you understand his concerns and objectives.
Explain that a court order is required to release the patient's information.

Interactive Case #9
Pharmacist – Standardized Physician Interaction

Your (Candidate) instructions:

Case description:

You are a pharmacist in a hospital pharmacy. Dr Russer is waiting in the pharmacy to discuss her patient's therapeutic regimen. Dr. Russer's patient Patrick Fung has been diagnosed with generalized seizures about 3 months ago. Patrick Fung has been taking lamotrigine for the past 3 months; he is already on a maintenance dose of 300 mg bid. Unfortunately, he is experiencing recurrent seizures. Dr. Russer would like to discuss with you if switching to another drug would be beneficial. You are expected to identify the best course of actions(s). Refer to the physician's introduction and questions, **below**, to fully understand her concerns and expectations.

This station must be completed in 7 minutes

Station materials and references: Compendium of Therapeutic Choices (CTC)

Patient profile

Name: Patrick Fung
Gender: Male
Age: 27 years old
Medical History: Generalized seizures diagnosed 3 months ago
Allergies: None
Current Medications (Rx & nRx): Lamotrigine 300 mg bid - missed scheduled refill
Social/lifestyle: Bar and night club musician, non-smoker, moderate alcohol intake – 3 to 5 drinks weekly, physically active – visits the gym at least 3 times a week

Standardized physician introductions and questions

"Hi, I am Dr. Russer. I am concerned about my patient's recurrent seizures. He has been on lamotrigine for the past 3 months but his condition is still not controlled. I would like to discuss switching him to another drug. What do you think about that?"

If the candidate suggests changing the medication, the standardized physician will ask:

"So, it means that lamotrigine is not effective in this patient. Do you have an explanation?"

Other questions:

"Is the new medication a drug of choice for monotherapy?"

"Should I take Patrick off lamotrigine before prescribing this medication?"

CASE REVIEW FORM

Write notes, answers, interview and counselling to show how you would solve this case

Solution – Interactive Case #9

<u>Primary goals</u>:

- Identify that, in this case, the recurrence of seizures is probably due to sleep starvation (bar and night club musician) and lack of compliance (the profile shows a missed scheduled refill). Alcohol reduction could be also beneficial.
- Recommend a re-counselling session.

You are expected to:

Identify that, in this case, the recurrence of seizures is probably due to sleep starvation (bar and night club musician) and lack of compliance; the profile shows a missed scheduled refill.

Recommend alcohol reduction. Alcohol interferes with the effectiveness of antiseizure drugs

Recommend a re-counselling session to re-educate the patient on the impact of poor compliance and lifestyle on the effectiveness of his therapeutic regimen

Explain that the usual maximum maintenance dose of lamotrigine is 400 mg, therefore increasing the dose should be considered first before switching to another drug

Explain if switching to another drug becomes appropriate in the future, she should add either phenytoin, valproic acid or carbamazepine then withdraw lamotrigine by tapering the dose. Lamotrigine, valproic acid, phenytoin and carbamazepine are drugs of choice for monotherapy.

Advise monitoring blood levels of lamotrigine.

Interactive Case #10
Pharmacist – Standardized Physician Interaction

Your (Candidate) instructions:

Case description:

Dr. David is waiting in the pharmacy to talk to you. She would like to discuss a new prescription for her patient Karyn Bob for the prevention of acute and delayed emesis. Karyn has been scheduled to be treated with cisplatin which is a highly emetogenic chemotherapeutic drug. You are expected to review the prescription and identify any drug related problem(s). Refer to the physician's introduction and questions, **below**, to fully understand her concerns and expectations. You are also expected to record your recommendations and any change(s) on the prescription review sheet.

Patient profile

Name: Karyn Bob
Gender: Female
Age: 47 years old
Medical History: Breast cancer – recently diagnosed
Allergies: Seasonal
Current Medications (Rx & nRx): 1 daily multivitamin, Tylenol prn for pain
Social/lifestyle: Non-smoker, no alcohol intake, physically active – gentle yoga 3 times a week

Station materials and references: Compendium of Pharmaceuticals and Specialties (CPS)
Compendium of Therapeutic Choices (CTC)

This station must be completed in 7 minutes

Prescription

```
                Getwell Hospital
                  5 Fall Road
                  Spring City
                   999-9999

For: Karyn Bob
Address: 344 Ottawa Blv

                                          Correct date


   Granisetron 1 mg prechemo and 12 h postchemo
   Lorazepam 1 mg prechemo, then 2 mg q4h prn
   Dexamethasone 10 mg prechemo, then 10 mg q12h

     L. David
   _____  Assume signature is correct
      L. David M.D.
```

Prescription Review Sheet

○ No change, fill the prescription as written

○ Recommended changes as discussed with Dr. David:

Correct date
Correct pharmacist's identification

Recommended dosage if required:

Standardized physician introductions and questions

"Hi, I am Dr. David. I have just written this new prescription for my patient Karyn Bob. What would you recommend regarding the prescription?"

If the candidate suggests changing the medication without explaining, the standardized physician will ask:

"Could you explain why?"

If the candidate recommends aprepitant, the standardized physician must ask:

"What will be the recommended dose for this drug?"

"Could you explain the mechanism of this drug?"

It the candidate fails to recommend a dose reduction of dexamethasone, the standardized physician will ask:

"Is there any likely interactions with the remaining drugs?"

CASE REVIEW FORM

Write notes, answers, interview and counselling to show how you would solve this case

Solution – Interactive Case #10

Primary goals:

- Recommend changing lorazepam to aprepitant.
- Identify aprepitant-dexamethasone interaction
- Recommend a lower dose of dexamethasone

The candidate is expected to:

- Recommend changing lorazepam to aprepitant (Emend).

- Recommend the following dosage of aprepitant (Emend):
125 mg orally 1 hour prior to chemotherapy treatment (Day 1) and 80 mg once daily in the morning on Day 2 and Day 3.

- Explain that based on clinical studies neurokinin-1 (NK1) antagonists such as aprepitant added to dexamethasone and a serotonin antagonist such as granisetron improve the prevention of acute **and** delayed emesis induced by highly emetogenic chemotherapy

- Benzodiazepines such as lorazepam are primarily used for anticipatory nausea.

- Explain that since aprepitant is a CYP3A4 inhibitor, it increases blood levels of dexamethasone. The dose of dexamethasone should not exceed 50% of the maximum dose of 10 mg. Change the dose of dexamethasone to 5 mg.

Interactive Case #11
Pharmacist – Standardized Physician Interaction

Your (Candidate) instructions:

Case description:

Dr Ali is waiting in the pharmacy to talk to you. He would like to discuss a new prescription for his patient Linda Thomas for the headaches. Her headaches typically range from moderate to severe. You are expected to review the prescription and identify any drug related problem(s). Refer to the physician's introduction and questions, **below**, to fully understand his expectations and concerns. You are also expected to record your recommendations and any change(s) on the prescription review sheet.

Patient profile

Name: Linda Thomas
Gender: Female
Age: 27 years old
Medical History: Migraine headaches– recently diagnosed
Allergies: None
Current Medications (Rx & nRx): 1 Materna multivitamin daily, Maalox prn
Social/lifestyle: Non-smoker, no alcohol intake, physically active – gentle yoga 3 times a week

Station materials and references: Compendium of Pharmaceuticals and Specialties (CPS)
Compendium of Therapeutic Choices (CTC)

This station must be completed in 7 minutes

Prescription

Sunny Hospital
200 High Road
Rainy City
888-9970

For: Linda Thomas
Address: 88-4th Avenue

                                                                                                    Correct date

Ergotamine
2 mg at onset of headache then 1 mg q1h prn x 3 doses

L. Ali
_____ Assume signature is correct
L. Ali M.D.

Prescription Review Sheet

○ No change, fill the prescription as written

○ Recommended changes as discussed with Dr. Ali:

Correct date
Correct pharmacist's identification

Recommended dosage if required:

Standardized physician introductions and questions

If asked, the physician will provide the following additional information:

Lynda had a baby girl 5 months ago and she is breastfeeding.

Important Note: The use of Materna (refer to profile) must prompt this investigation on your behalf. If you fail to ask, this key information will not be provided.

"Hi, I am Dr. Ali. I have just written this new prescription for my patient Linda Thomas. What you would recommend regarding the prescription?"

If the candidate suggests changing the medication without explaining, the standardized physician will ask:

"Could you explain why?"

If the candidate recommends an analgesic such as Tylenol, the standardized physician will ask:

"I would like to remind you that her headaches are moderate to severe. Do you think an analgesic will be effective?"

If the candidate recommends a triptan (e.g. sumatriptan, naratriptan), the standardized physician will ask:

"I am not familiar with this medication in my practice. Could you explain the mechanism of the drug? How about side effects? Which of the triptans has the highest safety profile?"

"What will be the dosage?"

It the candidate fails to warn about the potential of rebound headaches, the standardized physician will ask:

"Is there anything else I should know regarding the use of this drug?"

CASE REVIEW FORM

Write notes, answers, interview and counselling to show how you would solve this case

Solution – Interactive Case #11

<u>Primary goals</u>:

- Determine that the patient is a new mom who is breastfeeding
- Recommend changing ergotamine
- Explain that ergotamine could suppress lactation and have adverse effects on the child

The candidate is expected to:

Recommend changing ergotamine. Ergotamine could suppress lactation. Ergotamine is also excreted in breast milk which can potentially have adverse effects on the child.

Explain that since her headaches are moderate to severe, a triptan will be the best option. Naratriptan has the best safety profile among triptans and the lowest onset of action peak among triptans. Peak efficacy at 4 hours.

Explain that triptans are abortive drugs and serotonin receptor agonists. They are effective in the treatment of migraine and cluster headaches. However, using triptans for more than 10 days per month results in rebound headaches. Side effects include chest discomfort, fatigue, dizziness, paresthesia (pins and needles sensation) and nausea

Recommend the following naratriptan dosing:

1 to 2.5 mg ; may repeat in 4 hours. Max of 5 mg within 24 hours.

Interactive Case #12
Pharmacist – Standardized Physician Interaction

Your (Candidate) instructions

Case description:

Dr. Carlson is waiting in the pharmacy to talk to you regarding her patient's therapeutic regimen. Dr. Carlson's patient Jim Smith has been diagnosed with depression about 2 months ago. Jim Smith has been taking fluoxetine 40 mg daily for 8 weeks. Unfortunately, he is still experiencing persistent insomnia and anxiety. Dr. Carlson would like to discuss optional add-on drugs to improve therapeutic effectiveness. You are expected to recommend proven effective add-on drugs. Refer to the physician's introduction and questions, **below**, to fully understand her expectations and concerns.

Station materials and references: Compendium of Therapeutic Choices (CTC)

This station must be completed in 7 minutes

Patient profile

Name: Jim Smith
Gender: Male
Age: 30 years old
Medical History: Depression diagnosed 2 months ago
Allergies: None
Current Medications (Rx & nRx): Fluoxetine 40 mg daily x 8 weeks
Social/lifestyle: Hot yoga instructor, non-smoker, moderate alcohol intake – 5 to 8 drinks weekly

Standardized physician introductions and questions

"Hi, I am Dr. Carlson. My patient Jim is currently on fluoxetine for depression. Unfortunately, he is still experiencing persistent insomnia and anxiety. I would like to discuss optional add-on drugs to improve his condition. What would you suggest?"

If the candidate suggests a drug other than olanzapine, risperidone or quetiapine, the standardized physician will ask:

"Is this drug proven to be effective in the treatment resistant depression with persistent insomnia and anxiety?"

If the candidate fails to warn about the reduction of the regulation of body temperature, the standardized physician will ask:

"Is there anything else I should know about the use of the drug based on Jim's profile?"

If the candidate fails to recommend alcohol reduction, the standardized physician will ask:

"Is sedation likely with this drug?"

CASE REVIEW FORM

Write notes, answers, interview and counselling to show how you would solve this case

Solution – Interactive Case #12

<u>Primary goals</u>:

Recommend adding an antipsychotic drug. The atypical antipsychotics olanzapine, risperidone and quetiapine have been proven effective as add-on drugs in the management of treatment resistant depression with persistent insomnia and anxiety.

The candidate is expected to:

- Identify that the patient has treatment resistant depression.

- Recommend adding an antipsychotic drug. The atypical antipsychotics olanzapine, risperidone and quetiapine have been proven effective as add-on drugs in the management of treatment resistant depression with persistent insomnia and anxiety.

- Recommend alcohol reduction due to sedating effect of antipsychotics

- Warn that olanzapine, risperidone and quetiapine reduce the regulation of body temperature. Jim is a hot yoga instructor

Interactive Case #13
Pharmacist – Standardized Physician Interaction

Your (Candidate) instructions:

Case description:

Dr. Kim is waiting in the pharmacy to talk to you, the pharmacist on duty in a hospital pharmacy. He would like to discuss a new prescription for his patient Paul Sam for the prevention of diabetes. You are expected to review the prescription and identify any drug related problem(s). Refer to the physician's introduction and questions, below, to fully understand his expectations and concerns. You are also expected to record your recommendations and any change(s) on the prescription review sheet.

Station materials and references: Compendium of Pharmaceuticals and Specialties (CPS) Compendium of Therapeutic Choices (CTC)

This station must be completed in 7 minutes

Patient profile

Name: Paul Sam
Gender: Male
Age: 57 years old
Medical History: COPD, one episode of lactic acidosis 7 months ago, hyperlipidemia, prediabetes– recently diagnosed
Allergies: None
Current Medications (Rx & nRx): Salbutamol 2 puffs tid prn, tiotropium 18 ug inhaled daily, atorvastatin 40 mg daily
Social/lifestyle: Non-smoker, no alcohol intake, he has been on low fat diet since his hyperlipidemia diagnosis, physically active – 4 times a week

Prescription

Honeydew Clinic
77 Spring Street
Canada City
999-7777

For: Paul Sam
Address: 4555-10th Avenue

                                                                       Correct date

Metformin
100 mg divided bid x 3 months

R. Kim

_____ Assume signature is correct
R. Kim M.D.

Prescription Review Sheet

○ No change, fill the prescription as written

○ Recommended changes as discussed with Dr. Kim:

Correct date
Correct pharmacist's identification

Recommended dosage if required:

Standardized physician introductions and questions

"Hi, I am Dr. Kim. I have just written this new prescription for my patient Paul Sam. What you would recommend regarding the prescription?"

If the candidate suggests changing the medication without explaining, the standardized physician will ask:

"Could you explain why?"

"What are alternative drugs for the prevention of diabetes in high-risk patients?"

"Based on my patient's profile, what would you recommend?"

If the candidate suggests switching to acarbose, the standardized physician must ask:

"Could you explain the mechanism of action of acarbose?"

"I have more experience with metformin. How effective is acarbose compared to metformin?"

"What is the dosage of acarbose? How about side effects?"

CASE REVIEW FORM

Write notes, answers, interview and counselling to show how you would solve this case

Solution – Interactive Case #13

Primary goal:

Recommend changing metformin due to the patient's history of lactic acidosis.

The candidate is expected to:

- Recommend changing metformin. Metformin is contraindicated in patients with history of lactic acidosis.

- Explain that lactic acidosis is one of the side effects of metformin therefore is should not be used in patients with history of lactic acidosis. The following diseases increase the risk of lactic acidosis: AIDS, cancer, kidney failure, respiratory failure (asthma, COPD) and sepsis.

- Explain that acarbose, orlistat and thiazolidinediones (rosiglitazone and pioglitazone) are alternative drugs for the prevention of type 2 diabetes in high-risk patients.

- Recommend acarbose. Orlistat would be not/less effective in this patient who is already on low fat diet. TZDs have cardiovascular side effects and increase blood lipids. The rates of reduction of the progression from prediabetes to diabetes for metformin and acarbose are respectively 31% and 30%.

- Explain that acarbose inhibits intestinal alpha-glucosidase which reduces the digestion of carbohydrates and postprandial blood glucose levels. Acarbose does not cause hypoglycemia or weight gain. Its adverse effects are GI related including flatulence, diarrhea, abdominal pain and nausea. Acarbose is contraindicated in irritable bowel syndrome and inflammatory bowel disease.

- Recommend the following dosage: 50 – 100 mg tid with each meal; start low and go slow to minimize adverse effects.

Interactive Case #14
Pharmacist – Standardized Nurse Interaction

Your (Candidate) instructions

Case description:

Mrs. Cairns, an emergency room nurse, is waiting in the pharmacy to talk to you, the pharmacist on duty in a hospital pharmacy. They have just admitted a 3 years old patient who is dehydrated. Mrs Cairns is seeking your assistance to determine the volume of oral Pedialyte required for rehydrating the child. She is also expecting a recommendation of oral rehydration rate. The young patient has the following symptoms:

8% reduction of body weight. His predehydration weight was 10 kg.
Dry mucous membrane
Decreased production of tears
Marked reduction urine output
Slight increase in pulse
Normal blood pressure
His lab test shows serum Na+ level of 140 mmol/l and slight reduction of BUN/creatinine ratio

Refer to the nurse's introduction and questions, below, to understand her expectations and concerns. The candidate may interact with the physician to obtain additional information and clarify any concern(s).

A patient profile is not available.

Station materials and references: Compendium of Pharmaceuticals and Specialties (CPS)
Compendium of Therapeutic Choices (CTC)

This station must be completed in 7 minutes

Standardized nurse introductions and questions

"Hi, I am Mrs. Cairns, a nurse in the emergency room. I have a 3 years old patient who is suffering from dehydration. Could you calculate the volume of oral Pedialyte needed for rehydration? What will be the appropriate rate of dehydration?"

CASE REVIEW FORM

Write notes, answers, interview and counselling to show how you would solve this case

Solution – Interactive Case #14

<u>Primary goals</u>:

- Determine that the child is suffering from moderate isonatremic dehydration
- Calculate the fluid deficit
- Recommend appropriate rehydration rate

The candidate is expected to:

Determine that he child is suffering from moderate isonatremic dehydration. Isonatremic dehydration is the most common type of dehydration (80% of all cases) and is characterized by serum Na+ levels in the range of 130 – 150 mmol/l.

Calculate the fluid deficit using the formula:

Fluid deficit (l) = predehydration weight (kg) – present weight (kg)

Volume of pedialyte (l) = 10 kg – 9.2 kg = 0.8 l = 800 ml

For moderate isonatremic dehydration, the rate of rehydration is:

50 ml/kg over the first 4 hours then replace the remaining fluid deficit over the next 6 to 8 hours

Recommend 500 ml over the first 4 hours and the remaining 300 ml over the next 6 to 8 hours.

Interactive Case #15: Erythema
Pharmacist – Standardized Patient Interaction

Your (Candidate) instructions

Case description

A 34-year-old female with severe erythema and peeling of her face, shoulders, and arms is visiting the pharmacy to seek your advice on how to manage her condition. She has spent most of the previous day at an outdoor farmers' market. She stated that this was the worst sunburn she had ever experienced. Provide your assistance. Refer to the patient's introduction and questions to fully understand her expectations and concerns.

This station must be completed in 7 minutes

Station materials and references: Compendium of Pharmaceuticals and Specialties (CPS)

Patient profile

Patient Name: Anita Singh
Gender: Female
Age: 34 years old
Allergies: Seasonal
Medical History: Rheumatoid arthritis
Current medications (Rx & nRx): Methotrexate 15 mg po q week – dispensed 3 weeks ago,
Other: Advil prn for headaches, one daily multivitamin
Social/lifestyle: Non-smoker, no alcohol intake, physically active – visits the gym 5 times a week

Standardized patient introductions and questions

Case description

A 34-year-old female with severe erythema and peeling of her face, shoulders, and arms is visiting the pharmacy to seek your advice on how to manage her condition. She has spent most of the previous day at an outdoor farmers' market. She stated that this was the worst sunburn she had ever experienced. She is confident you will help.

Patient profile

Patient Name: Anita Singh
Gender: Female
Age: 34 years old
Allergies: Seasonal
Medical History: Rheumatoid arthritis
Current medications (Rx & nRx): Methotrexate 15 mg po q week – dispensed 3 weeks ago,
Other: Advil prn for headaches, one daily multivitamin
Social/lifestyle: Non-smoker, no alcohol intake, physically active – visits the gym 5 times a week

"Hi, I am Anita. I have very bad sunburn. I was at the farmers' market yesterday. Could you tell me what kind of product will help? I have never had anything like that."

Are you saying that my arthritis cannot be treated?

CASE REVIEW FORM

Write notes, answers, interview and counselling to show how you would solve this case

Solution – Interactive Case #15

Primary goals:

- Determine that the patient is suffering from methotrexate-induced photosensitivity. Her symptoms and her lack of prior exposure to methotrexate are likely indicative of phototoxic reaction
- Refer the patient to her physician to discuss alternate therapy
- Recommend strategies to minimize photosensitive reactions (see below)
- Recommend topical products such as cool wet dressings, antipruritics or corticosteroids to provide some relief
- Recommend using Tylenol for headaches instead of Advil; NSAIDs increase the levels of methotrexate

The candidate is expected to educate the patient by providing an overview of photosensitive reactions:

Photosensitive reactions can be classified into two categories:

Phototoxic reactions. Ultraviolet (UV) light activates the photosensitizing drug to emit energy that may damage adjacent skin tissue resulting in an intensified sunburn with skin peeling. Phototoxicity is characterized by a rapid onset of erythema, pain, prickling, or burning sensation of areas exposed to the sun, with peak symptoms occurring 12-24 hours after the initial exposure. The hallmark of this reaction is the appearance of a sunburn-like reaction on areas of skin with the greatest exposure to sunlight. These reactions do not involve the immune system; therefore, prior exposure or sensitization to a drug is not necessary for this reaction to occur.
Factors influencing the intensity and incidence of drug-induced phototoxicity include:
- The concentration, absorption, and pharmacokinetics of the drug.
- The dose of sunlight (duration of exposure and spectrum of sunlight).

Photoallergic reactions. Drug induced photoallergy is less common than phototoxicity, and requires prolonged or prior exposure to the photosensitizing drug. As the name suggests, this type of reaction is immune mediated. UV light reacts with the drug to produce an immunogenic hapten resulting in cell mediated immune response resulting in a skin reaction. Photoallergic reactions are not dose dependent and are characterized by urticaria (called solar hives) with eczema-like dermatitis and erythema. Light exposed areas on the skin are the predominant location of the reaction. These eruptions usually disappear spontaneously upon removal of the offending drug.

Management and prevention of drug-induced photosensitivity:

If the patient's typical activities require a significant amount of time outdoors, the use of an alternative therapy should be considered. Short-term courses may require temporary limitations on activities, while chronic therapy may necessitate alterations in daily activities.
Use of "night-time" dosing strategies, when possible, allows for maximum drug absorption and distribution during the night, thus minimizing sun exposure.

Strategies to minimize the risk of these reactions:

Avoid direct UV exposure from natural sunlight as well as tanning beds. Especially avoid the sun between 10 a.m. and 3 p.m.

Wear sun-protective clothing when going outdoors. If possible, wear shirts with high collars and long sleeves, pants or a long skirt, socks and shoes, a wide-brimmed hat, and sunglasses.

Use a UV-A and UV-B combination sunscreen with at least SPF 15.

Mild reactions are treated with topical products such as cool wet dressings, antipruritics, and corticosteroids.

Reassure the patient that other effective medications are available. Her physician will determine the best course of action.

Summarize and assess patient understanding

Interactive Case #16: Ethic
Pharmacist – Standardized Patient Interaction

Your (Candidate) instructions

Case description:

Ms. Jane Park is a 25 years old former college student. She has been diagnosed with Guillain-Barre syndrome two years ago. Since then, her condition has deteriorated. She can no longer walk and is confined in a wheel-chair. Based on her physician's assessment, she will be most likely intubated and living on a respirator within 5 months due to progressive respiratory muscles failure. Guillain-Barre syndrome is a disorder affecting the peripheral nervous system; typical presentation of the disease involves ascending paralysis and weakness beginning in the feet and hands and migrating towards the trunk. Unlike disorders such as multiple sclerosis (MS) and Lou Gehrig's disease (ALS), Guillian-Barre does not, in general, cause nerve damage to the brain or spinal cord. The disease is usually triggered by an infection. Jane's Mom brought her to your pharmacy with a prescription for methylprednisolone. Her Mom gives you the prescription and warns that her daughter has decided to refuse all treatments. Provide your assistance as you would in practice. Refer to the patient's statement to fully understand her expectations and concerns.

This station must be completed in 7 minutes

Standardized patient statement

Yes, I don't want anything to do with any treatment! My decision is final. I can no longer achieve my dreams of being married and having a family. I was dreaming of becoming an elementary school teacher. I have suffered enough; I just want to end it.

My doctor has been great including all the nurses. Everybody is very nice to me. I am grateful for that. I can no longer live and keep thinking about becoming confined to a respirator.

I was a happy, active and independent child. Now I need help for everything. I can't even feed myself. I don't want to live like that. I do understand what will happen if I refuse treatment and I don't need counseling. I have just completed a 3-week counseling session. I have made my decision 6 months ago. I have taken enough time to discuss my decision with my family and our church priest. They want the best for me and respect my wish. I do believe in God and have faith in God. I used to go to church every Sunday. I think I am spiritual.

CASE REVIEW FORM

Write notes, answers, interview and counselling to show how you would solve this case

Solution – Interactive Case #16

The candidate is expected to:

Address the patient directly. Ms. Jane is an adult with the capacity to understand the pharmacist. Please, recall that Guillian-Barre does not, in general, cause nerve damage to the brain or spinal cord.

Confirm that she has decided to refuse all treatments.

Ask if the patient has discussed her decision with family members and/or if she is willing to have a family meeting

Ask about the patient's mental and emotional state. Depression may be a concern.

Ask if patient would be interested in counseling or other types of support

Ensure that the patient has been given sufficient information about her condition.

Ensure that the patient understands fully the consequences of the decision.

Confirm that patient has the right to refuse treatment.

Explain that you will inform her physician. The physician will determine if there are other options to help keep her comfortable.
Encourage her to discuss her decision with her physician.

State that she can change her mind.

Interactive Case #17: Ethic
Pharmacist – Standardized Client Interaction

Case description:

A paramedic, Mr. Joe Smith, is in a community pharmacy to talk to the pharmacist (you). Mr. Smith appeared anxious and very concerned. A car has been involved in a serious head-on collision. The woman on board identified as Jane Peter is injured and her husband, who was driving, has died instantly following impact. Fortunately, the paramedics found, on the car back seat, a drug prescription refill bottle and receipt from your pharmacy across the street. The head of the team, Mr. Smith is requesting access to Mrs. Jane Peter's profile to help provide first-aid care on their way to the hospital emergency room. How would you handle Mr. Smith's request.

CASE REVIEW FORM

Write notes, answers, interview and counselling to show how you would solve this case

Solution – Interactive Case #17

The candidate is expected to:

First, inquire about Mrs. Peter's health status. In case she is alert and able to communicate, the pharmacist must take the necessary action (e.g. crossing the street to talk to Jane) to have her consent to release the profile.

In case, Jane is not able to provide consent (e.g. she is unconscious) then the pharmacist must provide the profile to help save her life. By providing the profile, the pharmacist will follow the principle of beneficence. Alternatively, if possible, a family member can provide consent. Unfortunately, the only family member on site (husband) is unable to provide consent.

Give Mr. Smith access the Jane's profile

Document your interaction with Mr. Smith including his full name and identification.

CASE REVIEW FORM

Write notes, answers, interview and counselling to show how you would solve this case

Interactive Case #18: Ethic
Pharmacist – Standardized Pharmacist Interaction

Case description:

Nicole Dylan is your longtime colleague. You have been good friends for almost twelve years; she is like your big sister. Nicole told you confidentially that she has been making lot of mistakes lately, she is being very forgetful. Nicole is turning 58 in 2 months. She mentioned that her recent physical exam showed that she is in good. She thinks her forgetfulness is simply showing her age. She explains that her work is becoming very stressful because she is constantly worried about harming someone due to her forgetfulness.

CASE REVIEW FORM

Write notes, answers, interview and counselling to show how you would solve this case

Solution – Interactive Case #18

The candidate is expected:

First, comfort and provide support to Nicole. Reassure that she can always count on your support and friendship.

Reassure that she is not alone. Many aging professionals are feeling the impact of their age on the workplace. The Canadian workforce is aging.

Remind Nicole that the safety of patients must be a priority.

Encourage her to discuss the matter openly with the pharmacy manager. The manager could offer a different work assignment or another workable solution

Discuss the situation with the manager if Nicole decides not to disclose her shortcomings to the manager. Failure to do that will be against the principle of non-maleficence.
Resolving the issue will be also in the best interest of Nicole because a fatal mistake has major consequences. Nicole's lack of cooperation could jeopardize the safety of patients.

Interactive case #19: Headache
Pharmacist – Standardized Patient Interaction

Your (Candidate) instructions

Case description:

A patient is seeking your advice on the management of migraine headaches. She has been using Imitrex for the past 2 months. Unfortunately her condition is not well controlled despite the use of the maximum dose of 200 mg daily for at least 3 days weekly. She has recently noticed that her condition has worsened resulting in recurrent headaches. She is now considering adding Tylenol to her current medication regimen to hopefully get better results. The patient is anxiously looking forward to your advice. Refer to the patient's introduction and questions to fully understand her expectations and concerns.

This station must be completed in 7 minutes

Station materials and references:
Patient profile
Compendium of Therapeutic Choices (CTC)
Compendium of Products for Minor Ailments

Patient profile

Patient Name: June Kim
Gender: Female
Age: 35 years old
Allergies: None known
Medical History: Migraine headaches, GERD - controlled
Current medications (Rx & nRx): Imitrex 200 mg daily, one multivitamin daily
Social/lifestyle: Secondary school teacher, non-smoker, no alcohol use, physically inactive – enjoys running 3 times weekly

Standardized patient introductions and questions

Case description:

A patient is seeking your advice on the management of migraine headaches. She has been using Imitrex for the past 2 months. Unfortunately her condition is not well controlled despite the use of the maximum dose of 200 mg daily for at least 3 days weekly. She has recently noticed that her condition has worsened resulting in recurrent headaches. She is now considering adding Tylenol to her current medication regimen to hopefully get better results. The patient is anxiously looking forward to your advice.

Patient profile

Patient Name: June Kim
Gender: Female
Age: 35 years old
Allergies: None known
Medical History: Migraine headaches, GERD - controlled
Current medications (Rx & nRx): Imitrex 200 mg daily, one multivitamin daily
Social/lifestyle: Secondary school teacher, non-smoker, no alcohol use, physically inactive – enjoys running 3 times weekly

"Hi, I am June Kim. I have been using a medication for headaches for the past two months. It doesn't seem to work. I am using it at least 3 days per week. I would like to have your advice on adding Tylenol. Do you think I will finally feel better? How much Tylenol should I take?"

If not addressed by the candidate after 5 minutes, the standardized patient will ask the following questions:

"Do you know why my headaches have worsened?"

CASE REVIEW FORM

Write notes, answers, interview and counselling to show how you would solve this case

Solution – Interactive Case #19

Primary goals:

- Determine that the patient is suffering from medication-overuse headache.
- Refer the patient to her physician for further assessment and consideration for prophylactic treatment.

If asked, the standardized patient will provide the following additional information:

Her migraine headaches have worsened recently.

The candidate is expected to:

Identify that the patient is suffering from rebound or medication overuse headaches.

Explain that Imitrex should not be use more than 10 days a month.

Explain that reducing the use of the medication could help.

Reassure the patient that other treatment options are available.

Refer the patient to her physician for further assessment. Her physician would also determine if she is a good candidate for a prophylactic treatment.

Recommend having a headache diary which would help monitor the effectiveness of treatment.

Discuss the following headache management strategies: avoid triggers, apply ice or rest in a dark noise-free room.

Discuss other non-pharmacologic options such as relaxation techniques, acupuncture and cognitive behavioural therapy (CBT).

Summarize and assess patient understanding

Interactive case #20: Cancer Pain Management
Pharmacist – Standardized Patient Interaction

Your (Candidate) instructions

Case description:

A cancer patient is visiting your pharmacy with a new prescription for Duragesic 50 mcg/h. He is seeking your assistance on how to use the patch and what to expect. Refer to the patient's introduction and questions to fully understand his expectations and concerns.

This station must be completed in 7 minutes

Station materials and references:

Patient profile
Compendium of Pharmaceuticals and Specialties (CPS)

Patient profile

Patient Name: Rick Berny
Gender: Male
Age: 56 years old
Allergies: Seasonal
Medical History: Prostate cancer
Current medications (Rx & nRx): Tylenol 500mg q6h
New prescription: Duragesic 50 mcg/h q3days
Social/lifestyle: Quit smoking 3 years ago, stopped drinking 2 years ago, regular mild yoga and swimming -3 to 4 times weekly

Standardized patient introductions and questions

Case description:

A cancer patient is visiting your pharmacy with a new prescription for Duragesic 50 mcg/h. He is seeking your assistance on how to use the patch and what to expect.

Patient profile

Patient Name: Rick Berny
Gender: Male
Age: 56 years old
Allergies: Seasonal
Medical History: Prostate cancer
Current medications (Rx & nRx): Tylenol 500mg q6h
New prescription: Duragesic 50 mcg/h q3days
Social/lifestyle: Quit smoking 3 years ago, stopped drinking 2 years ago, regular mild yoga and swimming -3 to 4 times weekly

"Hi, I am Rick. I have a new prescription for pain medication. Could you explain how I should apply it? How often should I use apply? I am also concerned about swimming? Should I remove it before getting wet?"

No, I have not used any narcotic before.

CASE REVIEW FORM

Write notes, answers, interview and counselling to show how you would solve this case

Solution – Interactive Case #20

<u>Primary goal</u>:

- Confirm that Mr. Berny is a naïve patient who has not used an opioid previously
- Call the physician to discuss the prescription. Fentanyl patch is contraindicated in naïve patients. The patch is used only in patients who are already receiving a total daily of at least 60 mg morphine.

<u>Additional learning</u>: Overview of fentanyl patch

The patch provides long-lasting pain relief over a long period of time up to 72 hours. However, breakthrough pain is likely due to a delay of up to 20 hours before onset of action OR when the medication is wearing off. Breakthrough pain is commonly treated with morphine or fentanyl lozenges.

To apply the patch:

- Tear the pouch open. Remove the patch.
- Fill out the dating sticker. It will help ensure that the patch is applied according to schedule.
- Hold the patch by the edge. Peel back the liner and safely discard it.
- Apply the patch to a dry area on the chest or back above the waist or to the upper arm. Clip the hair close to the skin but do not shave.
- Press the patch firmly on the skin for 10 - 20 seconds. Make sure it is firmly attached.
- The application area should not be oily or irritated/damaged. If needed, use plain water, not soap to wash the area; then pat dry without rubbing.
- After applying the patch, rinse hands with water only, do not use soap.
- Avoid strenuous exercise that may increase body temperature while wearing the patch to avoid increasing the levels of the medication in blood.
- The patch should be removed after 3 days. Apply a new patch to a different body area following the same steps.
- If he forgets to replace the patch at the scheduled time, he must apply it as soon as he remembers. Do not apply a new patch while another one is in place.
- If the patch comes off, apply a new one.
- Avoid using soaps, oil, lotions, alcohol, or other products around the patch. They may irritate the skin.
- He can bath, shower, or swim then pat dry the application area. Do not rub the skin around the patch. Excessive rubbing can affect the rate of medication absorption.
- Dispose of used patches by folding the sticky side then flush down the toilet.
- The medication in fentanyl patches is contained in a gel between layers of the patch. If this gel leaks from the patch, remove the patch right away without touching the gel. If you do touch the gel, immediately wash the area with large amounts of clear water. Do not use soap, alcohol, or other cleansers.

Common adverse reactions: nausea, constipation (recommend a stool softener), drowsiness, irritation at the site of application.

Immediate medical assistance is required in case of:
- Respiratory depression
- Fever
- Confusion
- Hallucinations

Interactive case #21: Treatment of urinary tract infection (UTI)
Pharmacist – Standardized Patient Interaction

Your (Candidate) instructions

Case description:

A female patient who has been diagnosed with acute urinary tract infection is visiting you pharmacy to fill a prescription for SMX/TMP. She has been experiencing burning while urinating and the urge to urinate frequently. Patient had a rash while taking sumatriptan for the treatment of migraine headaches which required switching to Tylenol #2. She is also interested in learning about potential side effects of SMX/TMP. Please, provide your assistance. Refer to the patient's introduction and questions to fully understand her expectations and concerns.

This station must be completed in 7 minutes

Station materials and references:

Patient profile
Compendium of Therapeutic Choices (CTC)

Patient profile

Patient Name: Miriam Hassan
Gender: Female
Age: 28 years old
Medical History: Migraines
Current medications(Rx & nRx): Sumatriptan switched to Tylenol #2 prn due to rash, 1 tablet of One a Day Women multivitamin
New prescription: SMX/TMP 400/80mg 2 tablets po BID for 3 days
Social/lifestyle: Lawyer, non-smoker, moderate alcohol intake – 3 to 5 drinks weekly, physically active – visits the gym at least 3 times weekly

Standardized patient introductions and questions

Case description:

A female patient who has been diagnosed with acute urinary tract infection is visiting you pharmacy to fill a prescription for SMX/TMP. She has been experiencing burning while urinating and the urge to urinate frequently. Patient had a rash while taking sumatriptan for the treatment of migraine headaches which required switching to Tylenol #2. She is also interested in learning about potential side effects of SMX/TMP.

Patient profile

Patient Name: Miriam Hassan
Gender: Female
Age: 28 years old
Medical History: Migraines
Current medications(Rx & nRx): Sumatriptan switched to Tylenol #2 prn due to rash, 1 tablet of One a Day Women multivitamin
New prescription: SMX/TMP 400/80mg 2 tablets po BID for 3 days
Social/lifestyle: Lawyer, non-smoker, moderate alcohol intake – 3 to 5 drinks weekly, physically active – visits the gym at least 3 times weekly

"Hi, I am Miriam. I just got this new prescription from my doctor. It is my first time having this type of infection. I truly hope this medication will give me some relief. Could you also tell me what to expect?"

If asked, the patient will provide the following additional information:

Her symptoms include sensation of burning and urge to urinate.

If not addressed by the candidate, after 5 minutes the standardized patient must ask the following questions:

"I had a rash while on my first headache medication. Do you think I should expect that with this medication?"

CASE REVIEW FORM

Write notes, answers, interview and counselling to show how you would solve this case

Solution – Interactive Case #21

<u>Primary goal</u>:

The candidate is expected to:

Identify that the patient has sulfa allergy. Sumatriptan is a sulfonamide.

Identify that Sulfamethoxazole (SMX) is also a sulfonamide therefore not recommended in this patient. Explain her/his findings to the patient.

Reassure and advise the patient that her physician will be called to switch to another first line therapy: Trimethoprim (TMP) 100 mg po BID for 3 days. Nitrofurantoin 7 day-therapy is another option which may not suit this patient due to the incidence of headaches.

Discuss non-pharmacologic strategies for the prevention of UTIs:

- Drink lot of fluids. Add cranberry and blueberry juice in your diet.
- Wipe from front to back after going to the toilet.
- Avoid douching
- Avoid using vaginal deodorants and perfumes

Summarize and assess patient understanding

Interactive case #22: Proper use of inhaler
Pharmacist – Standardized Patient Interaction

Your (Candidate) instructions

Case description:

Mr. Young has been a long-time smoker. After few months of recurrent cough, he has been diagnosed with congestive obstructive pulmonary disease (COPD). He is coming to see the pharmacist (you) with a new prescription for Atroven HFA (Ipratropium). He is looking forward to learning from the pharmacist how to properly use his puffer. Refer to the patient's introduction and questions to fully understand her expectations and concerns.

This station must be completed in 7 minutes

Station materials and references: Patient profile; Compendium of Pharmaceuticals and Specialties (CPS); Compendium of Products for Minor Ailments
Atroven HFA

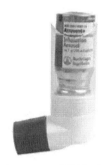

Atrovent HFA © Boehringer Ingelheim Inc.

Patient profile

Patient Name: Peter Young
Gender: Male
Age: 69 years old
Allergies: None
Medical History: Peptic ulcer, glaucoma
Current medications (Rx & nRx): Dorzolamide 1 drop Q8, 1 daily multivitamin, aspirin for occasional back pain
New prescription: Atroven HFA 2 puffs Q6 daily
Social/lifestyle: Retired, lives alone with family support, stopped smoking 3 years ago, no alcohol intake, enjoys swimming – 3 times weekly

Standardized patient introductions and questions

Case description:

Mr. Young has been a long-time smoker. After few months of recurrent cough, he has been diagnosed with congestive obstructive pulmonary disease (COPD). He is coming to see the pharmacist (you) with a new prescription for Atroven HFA (Ipratropium). He is looking forward to learning from the pharmacist how to properly use his puffer.

Patient profile

Patient Name: Peter Young
Gender: Male
Age: 69 years old
Allergies: None
Medical History: Peptic ulcer, glaucoma
Current medications (Rx & nRx): Dorzolamide 1 drop Q8, 1 daily multivitamin, aspirin for occasional back pain
New prescription: Atroven HFA 2 puffs Q6 daily
Social/lifestyle: Retired, lives alone with family support, stopped smoking 3 years ago, no alcohol intake, enjoys swimming – 3 times weekly

"Hi, I just got this new prescription from my doctor. It is my first time taking this medication and I am not sure how to use it properly. I am also wondering if I can use it if I have a sudden attack"

If not addressed by the candidate after 5 minutes, the standardized patient will ask the following questions:

"Can I use it if I have a sudden attack?"

"What should I do if I forget my medication?"

If asked, Mr. Young will provide the following additional information:

His glaucoma is well controlled with medication. He is no longer taking ulcer medication and has no symptoms.

If you fail to ask, this key information will not be provided. Therefore, knowledge of ipratropium adverse effects is important.

CASE REVIEW FORM

Write notes, answers, interview and counselling to show how you would solve this case

Solution – Interactive Case #22

Primary goals:

- Educate the patient on how to use the inhaler
- Recommend monitoring the patient's glaucoma
- Recommend Tylenol instead of aspirin for occasional back pain based on his history of peptic ulcer
- Ask about the status of his ulcer. Ipratropium could lead to worsening of ulcer.

The candidate is expected to:

Discuss the drug schedule with the patient. 2 puffs every 6 hours.

Explain how to use the Metered Dose Inhaler (MDI):
- Atroven HFA is a solution aerosol that does not require shaking
- Remove the cap
- Prime with 2 test sprays before first use. If the inhaler has not been used for more than 3 days, prime again by releasing 2 test sprays into the air away from the face.
- Breathe out, away from your inhaler
- Bring the inhaler to your mouth. Place it in your mouth between your teeth and close you mouth around it.
- Start to breathe in slowly. Press the top of you inhaler once and keep breathing in slowly until you have taken a full breath.
- Remove the inhaler from your mouth, and hold your breath for about 10 seconds, then breathe out.
- Wait 30s to 1 min before another puff. Repeat steps 3 to 6.
- Store the MDI at room temperature. If it gets cold, warm it using only your hands. When using a new MDI, write the start date on the canister. Check the expiry date on the MDI before use.
- Avoid contact with eyes to help minimize adverse effect on eye such as worsening of glaucoma. Recommend regular eye monitoring because the patient has glaucoma and to seek medical help immediately if vision changes
- Do not exceed 12 inhalations in 24 hours.
- The minimum interval between doses should not be less than 4 hours.

If you miss a dose, use it as soon as you remember it. If it is almost time for the next dose, skip the missed dose and carry on with regular schedule. Do not double a dose to make up for a missed one.

Discus common side effects: urinary retention, dry mouth, metallic taste (rinse mouth following drug administration)

Explain that Atroven HFA (Ipratropium) should not be used to treat sudden breathing problems where fast relief is needed. Fast acting medications (e.g., salbutamol, terbutaline) should be used for acute treatment. Refer the patient to his physician to determine if he needs such medication.

Discuss non-pharmacologic strategies:
- Avoid exposure to air pollution
- Physical activity helps improve symptoms

Recommend monitoring the patient's glaucoma
Recommend Tylenol instead of aspirin for occasional back pain based on his history of peptic ulcer
Ask about the status of his ulcer. Ipratropium could lead to worsening of ulcer.

Summarize and assess patient understanding

Interactive case #23: Omega-3 oil supplement
Pharmacist – Standardized Patient Interaction

Your (Candidate) instructions

Case description:

An elderly patient is visiting the pharmacy to seek the pharmacist's assistance to select an omega 3 oil supplement. A friend told him that omega-3 has several health benefits but he is still hesitant to take the product. He seems to be overwhelmed by the choices available and he is also concerned about proper dosage. He is confident that the pharmacist will help. Refer to the patient's introduction and questions to fully understand her expectations and concerns.

This station must be completed in 7 minutes

Station materials and references:

Patient profile
Natural Medicines Comprehensive Database
Cod fish oil – Omega-3, Vitamin A &Vitamin D bottle
Omega-3 EPA DHA 500 mg bottle

Patient profile

Patient Name: Joe Smith
Gender: Male
Age: 49 years old
Allergies: None
Medical History: Borderline type 2 diabetes managed with diet
Current medications (Rx & nRx): None
Other: Tylenol prn, one daily multivitamin
Social/lifestyle: Non-smoker, no alcohol intake, physically active – visits the gym 5 times a week

Standardized patient introductions and questions

Case description:

An elderly patient is visiting the pharmacy to seek the pharmacist's assistance to select an omega 3 oil supplement. A friend told him that omega-3 has several health benefits but he is still hesitant to take the product. He seems to be overwhelmed by the choices available and he is also concerned about proper dosage. He is confident that the pharmacist will help.

Patient profile

Patient Name: Joe Smith
Gender: Male
Age: 49 years old
Allergies: None
Medical History: Borderline type 2 diabetes managed with diet
Current medications (Rx & nRx): None
Other: Tylenol prn, one daily multivitamin
Social/lifestyle: Non-smoker, no alcohol intake, physically active – visits the gym 5 times a week

"Hi, could you tell me which one of these two products is best (refer to station materials)? A friend told me that omega-3 has many health benefits. I haven't used it yet. I am not sure how much will be enough. Could you help me with that?"

What kind of health benefits can I expect?

CASE REVIEW FORM

Write notes, answers, interview and counselling to show how you would solve this case

Solution – Interactive Case #23

Primary goals:

- Patient education. Provide an overview of omega-3 oil supplements.
- Recommend Omega-3 EPA DHA 500 mg instead of Cod fish oil

The candidate is expected to explain that:

Omega-3 fatty acids are a group of polyunsaturated fatty acids that are important for many body functions. Some studies have shown their beneficial effect in **diabetes**, rheumatoid arthritis, cardiovascular disease, depression, inflammatory diseases …They are found in fatty fish (e.g. salmon), certain vegetable oils (e.g. flax seed oil) and are also available in dietary supplements. Joe has borderline diabetes, make sure the highlight the potential benefit of omega-3.

Omega-3 fatty acid supplements usually do not have major negative side effects. When side effects do occur, they typically consist of minor gastrointestinal symptoms, such as belching, indigestion, or diarrhea.

Dosing for fish oil supplements should be based on the amount of EPA (Eicosapentaenoic Acid) and DHA (Docosahexaenoic Acid), not on the total amount of fish oil. Supplements have different amounts of EPA and DHA. The recommended dose is 1 gram daily of EPA and DHA combined.

Fish liver oils, such as cod liver oil, are not the same as fish oil. Fish liver oils contain vitamins A and D as well as omega-3 fatty acids. Both of these vitamins can be unsafe in large doses. Therefore, omega-3 EPA DHA 500 mg would be preferred. 2 capsules daily to get the recommended dose of 1 g EPA + DHA

Summarize and assess patient understanding

Interactive case #24
Pharmacist – Standardized Physician Interaction

Your (Candidate) instructions:

Case description:

You are working in a hospital pharmacy. Dr. Lam is waiting to see you with a new prescription for his patient Nancy Peter. You are expected to review the prescription and identify any drug related problem(s). You may interact with the physician to obtain additional information and clarify any concern(s). Record your recommendations and any change(s) on the prescription review sheet.

Station materials and references:

Handbook of Clinical Drug Data
Compendium of Pharmaceuticals and Specialties (CPS)
Prescription
Patient profile

This station must be completed in 7 minutes

Prescription

```
                    Wellness Hospital
                     5 Primary Road
                       Sunny City
                        666-6666

For: Nancy Peter
Address: 3 Ottawa Street

                                              Correct date

      Erythromycin
      500 mg QID x 10 days

        K. Lam
    _____     Assume signature is correct
        K. Lam M.D.
```

Patient profile

Name: Nancy Peter
Gender: Female
Age: 57 years old
Weight: 145 lbs
Medical History: Deep vein thrombosis (DVT), Pneumonia - just diagnosed
Allergies: Penicillin
Current Medications: Warfarin 5 mg daily - started 7 weeks ago

Additional information:

Nancy has been diagnosed with Streptococcus pneumoniae infection
Nancy's INR has been stable around 2.5. She has responded well to warfarin treatment. She will be using warfarin for at least 4 more weeks.

Prescription Review Sheet

○ No change, fill the prescription as written

○ Recommended changes as discussed with Dr. Lam:

Correct date
Correct pharmacist's identification

Recommended dosage if required:

Standardized physician introductions and questions

Case description:

Dr Lam is waiting in the pharmacy to talk to the pharmacist. He would like to discuss a new prescription for his patient Nancy Peter. The candidate is expected to review the prescription and identify any drug related problem(s). The candidate may interact with the physician to obtain additional information and clarify any concern(s). The candidate is also expected to record recommendations and any change(s) on the prescription review sheet. A patient's profile is provided.

Patient's profile

Name: Nancy Peter
Gender: Female
Age: 57 years old
Weight: 145 lbs
Medical History: Deep vein thrombosis (DVT), Pneumonia - just diagnosed
Allergies: Penicillin
Current Medications: Warfarin 5 mg daily - started 7 weeks ago

Additional information:

Nancy has been diagnosed with Streptococcus pneumoniae infection
Nancy's INR has been stable around 2.5. She has responded well to warfarin treatment. She will be using warfarin for at least 4 more weeks.

"Hi, I am Dr. Lam. I have just written this new prescription for my patient Nancy Peter. What you would recommend regarding the prescription?"

If the candidate suggests changing the medication without explaining, the standardized physician will ask:

"Could you explain why?"

If the candidate identifies a drug-drug interaction without explaining, the standardized physician will ask:

"What is the mechanism of this drug-drug interaction?"

If the candidate suggests changing the prescription to another medication other than **azithromycin**, the standardized physician will say:

"My previous patients have been successfully treated for Streptococcus pneumoniae infection using a macrolide therefore I would prefer prescribing a macrolide to Nancy. Could you recommend another macrolide?"

Once azithromycin is recommended by the candidate, the standardized physician will ask:

"What would be the dosage?"

CASE REVIEW FORM

Write notes, answers, interview and counselling to show how you would solve this case

Solution – Interactive Case #24

<u>Primary goals</u>:

- Identify and explain the mechanism to warfarin-erythromycin interaction
- Recommend an appropriate course of action to resolve the issue

Additional information:

Nancy has been diagnosed with Streptococcus pneumonia infection
Nancy's INR has been stable around 2.5. She has responded well to warfarin treatment. She will be using warfarin for at least 4 more weeks.

The candidate is expected to:

Identify warfarin-erythromycin interaction. Erythromycin is a potent inhibitor of CYP3A4 resulting in increased blood levels of CYP3A4 substrates such as warfarin. There is increased risk of bleeding. INR will increase.

Recommend azithromycin considering that a macrolide is preferred for this patient. The risk of interaction is minimal with azithromycin.

Explain that oral azithromycin given once a day for 5 days is equivalent to oral erythromycin given QID for 10 days. Once a day dosing is also likely to enhance compliance. Recommend the following dosage:

Azithromycin
500 mg po 1st day
Then 250 mg po daily for 4 days

Advise monitoring INR.

Interactive case #25
Pharmacist – Standardized Physician Interaction

Your (Candidate) instructions:

Case description:

You are working in a hospital pharmacy. Dr. Smith is waiting to see you with a new prescription for his patient James Park. You are expected to review the prescription and identify any drug related problem(s). You may interact with the physician to obtain additional information and clarify any concern(s). Record your recommendations and any change(s) on the prescription review sheet.

Station materials and references:

Handbook of Clinical Drug Data
Compendium of Pharmaceuticals and Specialties (CPS)
Patient profile
Prescription

This station must be completed in 7 minutes

Prescription

```
                    Hope Hospital
                    11 Spring Street
                    Main City
                    555-555

For: James Park
Address: 3- 22nd Drive

                                                    Correct date


        Fluoxetine
        20 mg daily x 30 days

           K. Smith
        _____      Assume signature is correct
           K. Smith M.D.
```

Patient's profile

Name: James Park
Gender: Male
Age: 50 years old
Weight: 220 lbs
Medical History: Parkinson's disease, Depression - newly diagnosed
Allergies: None Known
Current Medications: Selegiline 5 mg BID - started 3 months ago

Additional information:

Mr. Park has been just diagnosed with depression.
He has been on selegiline for the past three months and has responded well to treatment. His motor functions have improved.

Prescription Review Sheet

○ No change, fill the prescription as written

○ Recommended changes as discussed with Dr. Smith:

Correct date
Correct pharmacist's identification

Recommended dosage if required:

Standardized physician introductions and questions

Case description:

Dr. Smith is waiting in the pharmacy to talk to the pharmacist. He would like to discuss a new prescription for his patient James Park. The candidate is expected to review the prescription and identify any drug related problem(s). The candidate may interact with the physician to obtain additional information and clarify any concern(s). The candidate is also expected to record recommendations and any change(s) on the prescription review sheet. A patient's profile is provided.

Patient's profile

Name: James Park
Gender: Male
Age: 50 years old
Weight: 220 lbs
Medical History: Parkinson's disease, Depression - newly diagnosed
Allergies: None Known
Current Medications: Selegiline 5 mg BID - started 3 months ago

Additional information:

Mr. Park has been just diagnosed with depression.
He has been on selegiline for the past three months and has responded well to treatment. His motor functions have improved.

"Hi, I am Dr. Smith. I have just written this new prescription for my patient James Park. What you would recommend regarding the prescription?"

If the candidate suggests changing the medication without explaining, the standardized physician must ask:

"Could you explain why?"

If the candidate identifies a drug-drug interaction without explaining, the standardized physician will ask:

"What is the mechanism of this drug-drug interaction?"

If the candidate suggests changing the prescription to another medication other than **bupropion**, the standardized physician will say:

"So, this drug will not interact with selegiline. How about weight gain and sedation? I am concerned about Mr. Park's weight and his motor functions"

CASE REVIEW FORM

Write notes, answers, interview and counselling to show how you would solve this case

Solution – Interactive Case #25

<u>Primary goals</u>:

- Identify and explain the mechanism to selegiline - fluoxetine interaction
- Recommend an appropriate course of action to resolve the issue

The candidate is expected to:

Identify selegiline - fluoxetine interaction. Selegiline is an irreversible inhibitor of the enzyme monoamine oxidase B (MAO-B) which results in increased levels of fluoxetine leading to hypertensive crisis.

Recommend an antidepressant with a different mechanism of action that suits the patient. Mirtazapine leads to weight gain, Mr. Park weighs already 220 lbs. Trazodone is associated with excessive sedation at therapeutic doses, Mr. Park is already suffering from motor functions impairment. Bupropion would be the best option; it has a favorable side effect profile and low rate of sexual dysfunction.

Interactive case #26
Pharmacist – Standardized Physician Interaction

Your (Candidate) instructions:

Case description:

You are working in a hospital pharmacy. Dr. Hamid is waiting to see you with a new prescription for his patient Tim Scott. You are expected to review the prescription and identify any drug related problem(s). You may interact with the physician to obtain additional information and clarify any concern(s). Record your recommendations and any change(s) on the prescription review sheet.

Station materials and references:

Handbook of Clinical Drug Data
Compendium of Pharmaceuticals and Specialties (CPS)
Prescription
Patient Profile

This station must be completed in 7 minutes

Prescription

```
                    Grand Hospital
                    10 Seaview Street
                    Windy City
                    888-888

For: Tim Scott
Address: 882 Montreal Drive

                                              Correct date

        Sildenafil
        50 mg 30 to 60 min before sexual activity
        Mitte: 30 tablets

          R. Hamid
        _____   Assume signature is correct
            R. Hamid M.D.
```

Patient's profile

Name: Tim Scott
Gender: Male
Age: 49 years old
Weight: 175 lbs
Medical History: Peptic Ulcer, Erectile Dysfunction – just diagnosed
Allergies: None known
Current Medications: Cimetidine 300 mg qid - started 3 months ago

Additional information:

Tim has been diagnosed with peptic ulcer three months ago. He is currently on a maintenance dose of cimetidine.

Prescription Review Sheet

○ No change, fill the prescription as written

○ Recommended changes as discussed with Dr. Hamid:

Correct date
Correct pharmacist's identification

Recommended dosage if required:

Standardized physician introductions and questions

Case description:

Dr Hamid is waiting in the pharmacy to talk to the pharmacist. He would like to discuss a new prescription for his patient Tim Scott. The candidate is expected to review the prescription and identify any drug related problem(s). The candidate may interact with the physician to obtain additional information and clarify any concern(s). The candidate is also expected to record recommendations and any change(s) on the prescription review sheet. A patient's profile is provided.

Patient's profile

Name: Tim Scott
Gender: Male
Age: 49 years old
Weight: 175 lbs
Medical History: Peptic Ulcer, Erectile Dysfunction – just diagnosed
Allergies: None known
Current Medications: Cimetidine 300 mg qid - started 3 months ago

Additional information:

Tim has been diagnosed with peptic ulcer three months ago. He is currently on a maintenance dose of cimetidine.

"Hi, I am Dr. Hamid. I have just written this new prescription for my patient Tim Scott. What would you recommend regarding the prescription?"

If the candidate suggests changing the medication without explaining, the standardized physician will ask:

"Could you explain why?"

If the candidate identifies a drug-drug interaction without explaining, the standardized physician will ask:

"What is the mechanism of this drug-drug interaction?"

If the candidate suggests changing the prescription to another medication, the standardized physician will ask:

"As you know, sildenafil is effective and has a good safety profile. I would prefer prescribing it to Tim. Is there a way to use sildenafil and avoid this problem?"

If the candidate suggests changing cimetidine, the standardized physician will say:

"Tim has responded well to cimetidine and he is already on a maintenance dose. I would prefer not switching to another drug."

CASE REVIEW FORM

Write notes, answers, interview and counselling to show how you would solve this case

Solution – Interactive Case #26

Primary goals:

- Identify and explain the mechanism of cimetidine-sildenafil interaction
- Recommend an appropriate course of action to resolve the issue

The candidate is expected to:

Identify cimetidine-sildenafil interaction. Cimetidine reduces the metabolism of sildenafil resulting in more than normal blood levels (increased bioavailability). The risk of adverse reactions including hypotension is increased significantly.

This interaction can be managed by providing low dose of sildenafil, 25 mg instead of 50 mg as prescribed.

Interactive case #27: Social Anxiety
Pharmacist – Standardized Patient Interaction

Your (Candidate) instructions

Case description:

A female patient who has been recently diagnosed with social anxiety comes to see you with a new prescription for fluoxetine. She has some questions and concerns regarding the use of the medication. It is her first prescription for fluoxetine. Please, provide your assistance.

This station must be completed in 7 minutes

Station materials and references:

Patient profile
Compendium of Pharmaceuticals and Specialties (CPS)

Patient profile

Patient Name: Jane Peter
Gender: Female
Age: 28 years old
Allergies: None known
Medical History: Social anxiety diagnosed 5 days ago
Current medications (Rx & nRx): Advil prn for headaches
New prescription: Fluoxetine capsule 20 mg once daily

Note: The standardized patient shows some signs of shyness including avoidance of eye contact.

Standardized patient introductions and questions

Case description:

A female patient who has been recently diagnosed with social anxiety comes to see the pharmacist with a new prescription for fluoxetine. She has some questions and concerns regarding the use of the medication. It is her first prescription for the medication.

Patient profile

Patient Name: Jane Peter
Gender: Female
Age: 28 years old
Allergies: None known
Medical History: Social anxiety
Current medications (Rx & nRx): Advil prn for headaches
New prescription: Fluoxetine capsule 20 mg daily

"Hi, I just got this new prescription from my physician. It is my first time taking this medication and I am not sure how to use it. Could you also tell me what to expect?"

Note: the standardized patient shows some signs of shyness including avoidance of eye contact.

If asked, the patient will provide the following additional information:

Social/lifestyle: School bus driver, non-smoker, moderate alcohol intake – 3 to 5 drinks weekly

If not addressed by the candidate after 4 minutes, the standardized patient will ask the following questions:

What should I expect while taking this medication? Should I be concerned about grogginess?

What should I do if I forget my medication?

Should I see my doctor if I don't feel better in two weeks?

CASE REVIEW FORM

Write notes, answers, interview and counselling to show how you would solve this case

Solution – Interactive Case #27

<u>Primary goals:</u>

- Discuss the likelihood of drowsiness with regard to her occupation and alcohol consumption
- Discuss the relationship between NSAIDs and GI bleeding, and then recommend Tylenol instead.

The candidate is expected to:

Explain how to take the medication: Take one capsule once daily.
Discuss the common side effects of fluoxetine including agitation and drowsiness (at initiation of therapy), nausea, anorgasmia, dry mouth, insomnia, headache, decreased appetite, diarrhea, increased risk of GI bleeding. Recommend using fluoxetine in the morning (ideally at the same time) to reduce the likelihood of insomnia.

Discuss the incidence of drowsiness with regard to her occupation. She should avoid driving until she knows how the drug affects her. Warn that alcohol increases the incidence of drowsiness.

Recommend using Tylenol instead of Advil to manage headaches. NSAIDs increase the risk GI bleeding.

Explain that it may take 4 to 5 weeks before experiencing the full benefit of fluoxetine.
Advise the patient not to stop taking the medication without talking to her physician otherwise she may experience withdrawal symptoms such as mood changes, irritability, agitation, dizziness, numbness or tingling in the hands or feet, anxiety, confusion, headache, tiredness, and difficulty falling asleep or staying asleep. A gradual dose reduction would be required.

Educate the patient on missed dose management: take the missed dose as soon as you remember it. However, if it is almost time for the next dose, skip the missed dose and continue regular dosing schedule. Do not take a double dose to make up for a missed one.

Discuss non-pharmacologic options such as reduction of the intake of caffeine and other stimulants, stress reduction and relaxation techniques.

Summarize and confirm that patient understands

Interactive case #28: Insomnia
Pharmacist – Standardized Patient Interaction

Your (Candidate) instructions

Case description:

Mr. Smith is a young professional in his late twenties. He just moved in a new apartment building. He is visiting the pharmacy to purchase a nonprescription medication for the treatment of insomnia. He is seeking the pharmacist's assistance. Help the patient as you would in practice.

Note: The standardized patient shows signs of exhaustion due to lack of sleep.

This station must be completed in 7 minutes

Station materials and references:

Compendium of Products for Minor Ailments
Non-prescription medications: Nytol and Unisom
There is no patient profile

Standardized patient introductions and questions

<u>Case description</u>:

Mr. Smith is a young professional in his late twenties. He just moved in a new apartment building. He is visiting the pharmacy to purchase a non-prescription medication for the treatment of insomnia. Mr. Smith is seeking the pharmacist's assistance.

<u>Note</u>: The standardized patient shows signs of exhaustion due to lack of sleep.

"Hi, could you tell me which one of these medications would be best for my insomnia? I am a little confused."

There is no patient profile in the station. If asked, Mr. Smith will provide the following information:

Patient Name: Jim Smith
Age: 27 years old
Allergies: None
Medical History: None
Current medications (Rx & nRx): None
Social/lifestyle: Smoker – ½ pack daily, 3 to 4 alcoholic drinks weekly

He just moved in a new apartment building close to downtown. The neighborhood is quite noisy and the building does not seem to have good noise insulation.

He would like the pharmacist's help to select a nonprescription medication for insomnia. 2 nonprescription medications are available in the station.

CASE REVIEW FORM

Write notes, answers, interview and counselling to show how you would solve this case

Solution – Interactive case #28

<u>Primary goals</u>:

- Interview the patient to determine the cause of his insomnia
- Recommend ear plugs instead of a pharmacologic option

Patient profile (There is no patient profile in this station. The patient will provide the following information if requested)

Patient Name: Jim Smith
Age: 27 years old
Allergies: None
Medical History: None
Current medications (Rx & nRx): None
Social/lifestyle: Smoker – ½ pack daily, 3 to 4 alcoholic drinks weekly

He just moved in a new apartment building close to downtown. The neighborhood is quite noisy and the building does not seem to have good noise insulation.

The candidate is expected to:

Interview the patient and identify that the noisy neighborhood is most likely the primary reason of his insomnia.
Recommend the use of ear plugs instead of a nonprescription medication
Discuss other non-pharmacologic options such as regular exercise, avoid of stimulants and smoking (Jim is a smoker) in the evening, sleep in a dark room, avoid daytime napping, warm bath…
Counsel the patient on the benefits of stop smoking
Discuss smoking cessation strategies (nicotine replacement options) including non-pharmacologic options (social support, counselling)
Summarize and confirm patient understands

Interactive case #29: Antacid
Pharmacist – Standardized Patient Interaction

Your (Candidate) instructions

Case description:

A female patient is seeking your assistance to select an antacid to manage occasional heartburn. She had experienced few episodes of diarrhea with her previous antacid; unfortunately, she does not recall which antacid she had used. She seems to be overwhelmed by the different types of antacids available. Please, provide your assistance.

This station must be completed in 7 minutes

Station materials and references:

Patient's profile
Compendium of Products for Minor Ailments

OTC antacids:
Alka Seltzer
Maalox liquid
Milk of Magnesia
Pepto-Bismol

Patient profile

Patient Name: Marie John
Gender: Female
Age: 67 years old
Allergies: Aspirin
Medical History: Hypertension, postherpetic neuralgia
Current medications (Rx & nRx): Hydrochlorothiazide 25 mg once a day, Gabapentin 300 mg tid, Tylenol prn for headaches
Social/lifestyle: Non-smoker, No alcohol consumption, physically active – daily 35 minutes' walk

Standardized patient introductions and questions

Case description:

A female patient is seeking the pharmacist's assistance to select an antacid to manage occasional heartburn. She had experienced few episodes of diarrhea with her previous antacid; unfortunately, she does not recall which antacid she had used. She seems to be overwhelmed by the different types of antacids available.

Patient profile

Patient Name: Marie John
Gender: Female
Age: 67 years old
Allergies: Aspirin
Medical History: Hypertension, postherpetic neuralgia
Current medications (Rx & nRx): Hydrochlorothiazide 25 mg once a day, Gabapentin 300 mg tid, Tylenol prn for headaches
Social/lifestyle: Non-smoker, No alcohol consumption, physically active – daily 35 minutes walk

"Hi, could you tell me which of these products is best for my heartburns? I had diarrhea with one of them but I don't remember which one. I am just looking for something that works for me. Could you help me?"

4 OTC medications are available in the station.

If not addressed by the candidate after 4 minutes, the standardized patient will ask:

"Can I use it with my other medications?"

"Should I expect to have diarrhea again?"

CASE REVIEW FORM

Write notes, answers, interview and counselling to show how you would solve this case

Solution – Interactive Case #29

Primary goals:

- Identify the antacid linked to diarrhea (Mg containing product such as Milk of Magnesia)
- Recommend Maalox because it contains both Mg (diarrhea inducer) and Alu (constipation inducer) which provides a good balance
- Avoid Na containing products such as Alka Seltzer due to possible adverse effect on hypertension
- Avoid aspirin containing Pepto-Bismol due to her aspirin allergy

The candidate is expected to:

Recommend Maalox

Explain why Alka Seltzer and Milk of Magnesia and Pepto-Bismol should be avoided

Discuss the interaction between antacid and gabapentin, and recommend taking Maalox at least 2 hours before taking gabapentin. Antacids reduce the absorption of gabapentin.

Congratulate and encourage the patient to continue staying active. Discuss the benefits of physical activity in hypertensive patients.

Recall other non-pharmacologic strategies in the management of hypertension such as weight loss and healthy diet.

Recommend the application of a washcloth dipped in cool water to help reduce shingles pain and dry the blisters.

Recommend stress reduction strategies such as relaxation techniques to help manage the pain.

Explain that good body hygiene helps reduce secondary bacterial infections.

Summarize and confirm that patient understands

Interactive case #30: Depression
Pharmacist – Standardized Patient Interaction

Your (Candidate) instructions

Case description:

A young female patient is visiting your pharmacy to fill a new prescription for the treatment of depression. She has been experiencing some feelings of unexplained deep sadness for several months. As a result of that she has dropped out of college. The patient has been recently diagnosed with depression. It is her first prescription for an antidepressant therefore she is expecting to learn about how to use the medication and what to expect. Please, provide your assistance.

This station must be completed in 7 minutes

Station materials and references:

Patient profile
Compendium of Therapeutic Choices (CTC)

Patient profile

Patient Name: Liz Park
Gender: Female
Age: 22 years old
Allergies: None known
Medical History: Anorexia two years ago. The condition was managed with family support and counseling for 3 weeks.
Current medications (Rx & nRx): None
New prescription: Wellbutrin SR 75 mg BID

Note: The standardized patient shows signs of sadness and fatigue.

Standardized patient introductions and questions

Case description:

A young female patient is visiting the pharmacy to fill a new prescription for the treatment of depression. She has been experiencing some feelings of unexplained deep sadness for several months. As a result of that she has dropped out of college. The patient has been recently diagnosed with depression. It is her first prescription for an antidepressant therefore she is expecting to learn about how to use the medication and what to expect.

Patient profile

Patient Name: Liz Park
Gender: Female
Age: 22 years old
Allergies: None known
Medical History: Anorexia two years ago. The condition was managed with family support and counseling for 3 weeks.
Current medications (Rx & nRx): None
New prescription: Wellbutrin SR 75 mg BID

"Hi, I just got this new prescription from my physician. It is my first time taking this medication and I am not sure how to use it. Could you also tell me what to expect?"

Note: The standardized patient shows signs of sadness and fatigue.

If asked, the patient will provide the following additional information:

Social/lifestyle: College student, non-smoker, no alcohol use

She used to be anorexic. Her condition was managed with counselling and family support. Her weight is now normal.

CASE REVIEW FORM

Write notes, answers, interview and counselling to show how you would solve this case

Solution – Interactive Case #30

<u>Primary goals</u>:

- Identify that Wellbutrin (Bupropion) is contraindicated in patients with history of anorexia.
- Inform the patient that her physician will be contacted to change the medication.
- Reassure the patient that there are other effective optional treatments.

The candidate is expected to:

- Confirm that the patient has a history of anorexia

- Explain that bupropion is contraindicated in patient with a history of anorexia

- Reassure the patient that other effective treatment options are available

- Reassure the patient that her physician will be contacted to recommend another medication

- Discuss non-pharmacologic options such as cognitive behavioral therapy (CBT) and interpersonal psychotherapy (IPT). Her anorexia was managed with counselling and family support

- Summarize and assess patient understanding

Interactive case #31: Smoking Cessation
Pharmacist – Standardized Patient Interaction

Your (Candidate) instructions

Case description:

A male patient is visiting your pharmacy to ask for your advice regarding the use of nicotine patch to help him quit smoking. In the past, he has not been successful quitting without any nicotine replacement. He is fully committed and very optimistic about the outcome. He likes the discretion provided by the patch. Please, provide your assistance.

This station must be completed in 7 minutes

Station materials and references:

Patient's profile
Compendium of Therapeutic Choices (CTC)

Patient profile

Patient Name: Derek Ming
Gender: Male
Age: 32 years old
Allergies: Seasonal allergies
Medical History: None
Current medications (Rx & nRx): None
Social/lifestyle: Fitness instructor, smoker for 10 years – more than 1 pack daily, moderate alcohol intake – 3 drinks weekly.

His previous two attempts to stop smoking have not been successful. He is now considering a nicotine patch as stop smoking aid.

Note: The standardized patient shows signs of optimism and excitement about stop smoking.

Standardized patient introductions and questions

<u>Case description</u>:

A male patient is visiting the pharmacy to ask for your advice regarding the use of nicotine patch to help him quit smoking. In the past, he has not been successful quitting without any nicotine replacement. He is fully committed and very optimistic about the outcome. He likes the discretion provided by the patch.

Patient profile

Patient Name: Derek Ming
Gender: Male
Age: 32 years old
Allergies: Seasonal allergies
Medical History: None
Current medications (Rx & nRx): None
Social/lifestyle: Fitness instructor, smoker for 10 years – more than 1 pack daily, moderate alcohol intake – 3 drinks weekly.

"Hi, I would like to start using a nicotine patch to help me stop smoking. I have not been successful quitting without medication. I would like to keep my efforts private. Could you explain how to use it?"

<u>Note</u>: The standardized patient shows signs of optimism and excitement about stop smoking.

If asked, Mr. Ming will provide the following additional information:

His previous two attempts to stop smoking have not been successful. He is now considering a nicotine patch as stop smoking aid. He likes the discretion provided by the patch.

He is planning to stop smoking within 5 days.

If not addressed by the candidate after 4 minutes, the standardized patient will ask the following question:

"Can I use the patch while exercising? I'm a fitness instructor."

CASE REVIEW FORM

Write notes, answers, interview and counselling to show how you would solve this case

Solution – Interactive Case #31

Primary goals:

- Determine that the patch is not an appropriate nicotine replacement product for a fitness instructor who is regularly engaged in strenuous physical activities.
- Recommend nicotine gum instead of inhaler to respect the patient's need for discretion.
- Educate the patient on the use of nicotine gum

The candidate is expected to:

Reassure the patient that previous failures do not prevent future success.

Explain the five evidence-based steps required to stop smoking:

- Setting a target quit date
- Getting professional help
- Having social support
- Using medication such as nicotine replacement products
- Applying problem-solving strategies learned in counseling

Explain that nicotine replacement products help quit by easing nicotine withdrawal symptoms such as anger, anxiety, cravings, difficulty concentrating, hunger, impatience and restlessness. With nicotine replacement therapy, you can slowly lower your dose of nicotine as your body adjusts to being smoke-free.

Explain that the patch is not the appropriate option for him because his occupation leads to strenuous exercise which will increase the level of nicotine in blood leading to side effects.

Recommend nicotine gum instead. The inhaler is also unlikely to be a good option for someone who is concerned about discretion. The gum and inhaler give a more immediate effect of nicotine. Considering that the patient is a heavy smoker, recommend: 4 mg/piece

- 10 to 12 pieces/day initially to max of 20 pieces for 8 to 12 weeks then reduce by 1 piece daily each week as withdrawal symptoms allow.
- Then gradually decrease the total number of pieces used per day.
- Gradually replace 4 mg gum with 2 mg gum.
- Gradual reduction of chewing time from 30 minutes to 10 to 15 minutes is also a helpful dose reduction strategy.

Explain that nicotine gum should be chewed slowly until he can taste the nicotine or feel a slight tingling in his mouth. Then stop chewing and place the chewing gum between the cheek and gum. When the tingling is almost gone (usually within 1 minute), start chewing again. Repeat for about 30 minutes. Do not chew nicotine gum too fast, do not chew more than one piece of gum at a time, and do not chew one piece too soon after another. He should plan to stop using the gum when his craving for nicotine is satisfied by one or two pieces of gum per day.

Explain that smoking while using nicotine gum can cause the buildup of nicotine to toxic levels. Avoid smoking.

Recommend follow-up to monitor progress and provide encouragement.

Discuss common side effects: headaches, nausea and other GI problems, hiccoughs, jaw pain due to chewing

Discuss weight management strategies considering that here is potential weight gain following smoking cessation.

Summarize and assess patient understanding

Interactive case #32: Ginkgo
Pharmacist – Standardized Patient Interaction

Your (Candidate) instructions

Case description:

Mr. Singh is visiting the pharmacy located in a Shopping Mall to seek your advice regarding ginkgo. He learned from few friends that ginkgo can improve his memory. He is wondering if he should start using it. Mr. Singh is already taking two heart medications. Assist the client as you would in practice.

This station must be completed in 7 minutes

Station materials and references:

Natural Medicines Comprehensive Database
Compendium of Therapeutic Choices (CTC)
There is no patient profile

Standardized patient introductions and questions

Case description:

Mr. Singh is visiting the pharmacy located in a Shopping Mall to seek the pharmacist's advice regarding ginkgo. He learned from few friends that ginkgo can improve his memory. He is wondering if he should start using it. Mr. Singh is already taking two heart medications.

"Hi, I would like to have your advice regarding ginkgo. Do you think I should start using it to improve my memory? At least two of my friends are using it. I am thinking about adding it to my shopping list"

There is no patient profile in this station. If asked, Mr. Singh will provide the following information:

He is 65 years old.

At least two of his friends are taking ginkgo.

It is his first time visiting the pharmacy. He just decided to stop by because the location is convenient. His regular pharmacy is in a different location.

He can't tell exactly what kind of heart medications you are taking. He started taking both 4 years ago.

CASE REVIEW FORM

Write notes, answers, interview and counselling to show how you would solve this case

Solution – Interactive Case #32

<u>Primary goals</u>:

- Provide an overview of the potential health benefits of ginkgo
- Refer the client to his physician to assess his memory impairment and to determine if he can safely use ginkgo.

The candidate is expected **to some extent** to:

Explain that ginkgo is an herb. The leaves are used to make extracts that are used as medicine. Ginkgo works by improving blood circulation, which might help the functions of brain, eyes, ears, and legs.

Explain that studies have shown that ginkgo is possibly effective in:

- Alzheimer's disease and other forms of dementia.
- Improving thinking in young people.
- Raynaud's syndrome (high sensitivity to cold especially in fingers and toes.
- Claudication and peripheral vascular disease due to poor blood circulation.
- Vertigo and dizziness.
- Glaucoma.
- Improving color vision in people with diabetes.

Ginkgo is in general safe for most people. It can cause some minor side effects such as stomach upset, headache, dizziness, constipation, forceful heartbeat, and allergic skin reactions.

Warn that ginkgo interacts with many medications including (*this section may be limited to cardiovascular drugs only*):

Cytochrome P450 1A2 (CYP1A2) substrates (decreased metabolism, increased side effects) such as clozapine, cyclobenzaprine, fluvoxamine, haloperidol, imipramine, mexiletine, olanzapine, pentazocine, propranolol, tacrine, theophylline, zileuton, zolmitriptan, and others.

Cytochrome P450 2C19 (CYP2C19) substrates (increased metabolism, reduction of effectiveness) such as amitriptyline, citalopram, diazepam, lansoprazole, omeprazole, phenytoin, warfarin, and many others.

Cytochrome P450 2D6 (CYP2D6) substrates (decreased metabolism, increased side effects) such as amitriptyline, clozapine, codeine, desipramine, donepezil, fentanyl, flecainide, fluoxetine, meperidine, methadone, metoprolol, olanzapine, ondansetron, tramadol, trazodone, and others.

Cytochrome P450 3A4 (CYP3A4) substrates (increased side effects): lovastatin, clarithromycin, cyclosporine, diltiazem, estrogens, indinavir, triazolam, and others.

Diabetes medications (reduced effectiveness): glimepiride, glyburide, insulin, pioglitazone, rosiglitazone, chlorpropamide, glipizide, tolbutamide, and others.

Seizure threshold lowering drugs (increased risk of seizures): antiarrhythmics (mexiletine), antibiotics (amphotericin, penicillin, cephalosporins, imipenem), antidepressants (bupropion, others), antihistamines (cyproheptadine, others), immunosuppressants (cyclosporine), narcotics (fentanyl, others), stimulants (methylphenidate), theophylline, and others.

Anticoagulant / antiplatelet drugs (increased effectiveness): aspirin, clopidogrel, dalteparin, enoxaparin, heparin, indomethacin, ticlopidine, warfarin, and others.

Anticonvulsants (reduced effectiveness): phenobarbital, primidone, valproic acid, gabapentin, carbamazepine, phenytoin, and others.

Refer the client to his physician to assess his memory impairment (the risk of Alzheimer's is high around his age) and to determine if he can safely use ginkgo supplements.

Summarize and assess patient understanding

Interactive case #33: Shingles Pain
Pharmacist - Standardized Patient Interaction

Your (Candidate) instructions

Case description:

An elderly patient who has been recently diagnosed with shingles pain is visiting your pharmacy with a new prescription for famciclovir and amitriptyline. He went to see his physician following the sudden appearance of a painful rash on the left side of his trunk. He is seeking your advice on how to use the medications. He is also wondering why he needs two medications instead of one. Please, provide your assistance.

This station must be completed in 7 minutes

Station materials and references:

Patient profile
Compendium of Therapeutic Choices (CTC)

Patient profile

Patient Name: James Kim
Gender: Male
Age: 70 years old
Allergies: Seasonal allergies
Medical History: Type 2 diabetes, hyperlypidemia
Current medications (Rx & nRx): Metformin 500 mg tid, fenofibrate 160mg daily, one multivitamin daily, one omega-3 capsule
New prescription: Famciclovir 500 mg tab q8h for 7 days, amitriptyline 10 mg tab qhs increase by 10 mg daily at weekly intervals until pain relief
Social/lifestyle: Retired, non-smoker, no alcohol use, physically active – yoga classes and 30 minute-walk five times weekly

Standardized patient introductions and questions

Case description:

An elderly patient who has been recently diagnosed with shingles pain is visiting the pharmacy with a new prescription for famciclovir and amitriptyline. He went to see his physician following the sudden appearance of a painful rash on the left side of his trunk. He is seeking the pharmacist's advice on how to use the medications. He is also wondering why he needs two medications instead of one.

Patient profile

Patient Name: James Kim
Gender: Male
Age: 70 years old
Allergies: Seasonal allergies
Medical History: Type 2 diabetes, hyperlipidemia, shingles - newly diagnosed
Current medications (Rx & nRx): Metformin 500 mg tid, fenofibrate 160mg daily, one multivitamin daily, omega-3 supplement
New prescription: Famciclovir 500 mg tab q8h for 7 days, amitriptyline 10 mg tab qhs
Social/lifestyle: Retired, non-smoker, no alcohol use, physically active – yoga classes and 30-minute walk five times weekly

"Hi, I just got this new prescription from my physician. Could you tell me why I need two medications? I am not sure how to use them. Could you also tell me what to expect?"

If not addressed by the candidate, after 4 minutes, the standardized patient will ask the following questions:

"Why do I need both?"

"What should I expect while taking the medications? Should I be concerned about grogginess?"

"How should I use the two medications?"

CASE REVIEW FORM

Write notes, answers, interview and counselling to show how you would solve this case

Solution – Interactive Case #33

<u>Primary goal</u>:

Educate the patient.

The candidate is expected to:

Explain that his condition is due to the reactivation of the varicella zoster virus

Famciclovir is an antiviral medication. Amitriptyline is used to relieve pain.
Explain how to take the medications:
- Take 1 tablet of famciclovir every 8 hours for 7 days
- Take 1 tablet of amitriptyline at bedtime, increase by 1 tablet daily at weekly intervals until pain relief

Discuss the side effects of the medications:
Famciclovir: headache, somnolence, nausea, vomiting constipation
Amitriptyline: dry mouth, constipation, drowsiness, blurred vision, urinary retention, confusion, weight gain and tachycardia. Increase hydration to prevent dry mouth or use an artificial saliva spray. A stool softener can be used for constipation. Amitriptyline may color urine blue-green.

Summarize and assess patient understanding

Interactive case #34: Application of Eye Drops
Pharmacist – Standardized patient Interaction

Your (Candidate) instructions

Case description:

A young female patient is coming to see you regarding the proper application of nonprescription drops for dry eyes. She has been dealing with occasional dry eyes since she started using soft contact lenses 3 weeks ago. Her eye doctor has recommended the use of nonprescription Visine Dry Eye to ease her symptoms.

Please, provide your assistance.

This station must be completed in 7 minutes

Station materials and references:

Compendium of Pharmaceuticals and Specialties (CPS)
No patient profile
Visine Dry Eye

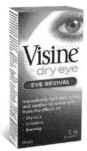

Visine Dry Eye © Johnson & Johnson Inc.

Standardized patient introductions and questions

Case description:

A young female patient is coming to see the pharmacist regarding the proper application of nonprescription drops for dry eyes. She has been dealing with occasional dry eyes since she started using soft contact lenses 3 weeks ago. Her eye doctor has recommended the use of nonprescription Visine Dry Eye to ease her symptoms.

There is no patient's profile in this station. If asked, the patient will provide the following information:

Patient Name: Susan Ali
Age: 23 years old
Allergies: None
Medical History: None
Current medications (Rx & nRx): None
Social/lifestyle: College student, non-smoker, occasional alcoholic drinks 1 to 2 weekly, plays basketball 4 times a week

She switched to contact lenses 3 weeks ago

She has been using prescription glasses for more than 5 years

Her symptoms include irritation, burning and some tearing

"Hi, I just got these eye drops my eye doctor has recommended. I am not sure how to use them properly. Could you help me with that? How many drops do I need?"

If not addressed by the candidate after 4 minutes, the standardized patient will ask:

"Do I have to remove my contact lenses before using the drops?"

CASE REVIEW FORM

Write notes, answers, interview and counselling to show how you would solve this case

Solution – Interactive Case #34

<u>Primary goal</u>:

Demonstration of the application of eye drops.

There is no patient profile in this station. If asked, the standardized patient will provide the following information:

Patient Name: Susan Ali
Age: 23 years old
Allergies: None
Medical History: None
Current medications (Rx & nRx): None
Social/lifestyle: College student, non-smoker, occasional alcoholic drinks 1 to 2 weekly, plays basketball 4 times a week

She switched to contact lenses 3 weeks ago

She has been using prescription glasses for more than 5 years

Her symptoms include irritation, burning and some tearing

The candidate is expected to:

Demonstrate and explain the proper application of eye drops:

- Before using eye drops, wash your hands with soap and warm water. Dry them with a clean towel.
- While tilting your head back, pull the lower lid of your eye down with one hand using two fingers to create a pocket. Hold the eye drops bottle in the other hand.
- Squeeze the bottle to place one eye drop inside your lower lid. The tip of the medication bottle should not touch your eye.
- Blink and dab away the excess eye drop fluid with a tissue.
- Keeping the eyes closed for a while may allow better penetration and effectiveness of the medication.
- Wait at least 5 minutes before placing another drop.
- Replace the cap on the bottle and wash your hands.

Place one to two drops as needed.

No need to remove contact lenses.

Advise the patient to avoid irritants such as wind, smoke or prolonged computer use.

Summarize and assess that patient understands.

Interactive case #35: Proper Use of Body Thermometer
Pharmacist – Standardized Client Interaction

Your (Candidate) instructions

Case description:

A 28 years old mom is visiting your pharmacy to seek the pharmacist's advice regarding the proper use of a body thermometer. Her daughter is 6 months old. Mrs. Jane Gill is a concerned mom who would like to be well prepared to take care of her baby. She has also learned in a magazine that temperature can be measured at different body sites.

This station must be completed in 7 minutes

Station materials and references:

Compendium of Products for Minor Ailments
There is no profile
Body thermometer

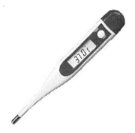

Note: The standardized client show signs of openness to learn from the pharmacist.

Standardized client introductions and questions

Case description:

A 28 years old mom is visiting the pharmacy to seek the pharmacist's advice regarding the proper use of a body thermometer. Her daughter is 6 months old. Mrs. Jane Gill is a concerned mom who would like to be well prepared to take care of her baby. She has also learned in a magazine that temperature can be measured at different body sites.

"Hi, I just got this body thermometer for my 6 months old baby. Could you explain how I should use it in case she has fever? I have also learned in a magazine that temperature can be measured at different body sites. Which body site will be best for my daughter? Also, what will be normal temperature?

Note: The standardized client show signs of openness to learn from the pharmacist.

If asked, she will provide the following additional information:

"It is my first child."

"She doesn't have fever; I just want to be prepared."

If not addressed by the candidate after 4 minutes, the client will ask the following questions:

"What temperature would be a sign of fever?"

"Which body site will be best for my daughter?"

CASE REVIEW FORM

Write notes, answers, interview and counselling to show how you would solve this case

Solution – Interactive Case #35

Primary goals:

- Educate the patient on the proper use of a body thermometer
- Recommend measuring rectal temperature
- Educate the patient on normal rectal temperature for a 6 months old infant

The candidate is expected to:

Explain that fever is a temporary increase in body temperature in response to some disease or illness. The most common cause of fever in children is an infection.

Confirm that mouth, rectum, armpit and ear are all optional body areas for measuring body temperature. However, the readings are slightly different.

Explain that rectal (at the bottom) body temperature is preferred for children younger than five years old because they are not able to maintain the thermometer safely either in the mouth or armpit.

Explain that electronic thermometers are the most recommended because the temperature is easily displayed and the probe can be placed in the mouth, rectum, or armpit.

Explain how to properly measure her daughter's temperature rectally:

- Place petroleum jelly on the bulb of a rectal thermometer.
- Place the small child face down on a flat surface or lap.
- Spread the buttocks and insert the bulb end about 1/2 to 1 inch into the anal canal. Be careful not to insert it too far.
- Remove after 3 minutes or when it beeps.
- Always clean the thermometer before and after use. Use cool, soapy water or rubbing alcohol
- After a warm bath, wait at least one hour before measuring body temperature.

Discuss that a child has fever when the temperature is at or above 38 °C measured in the bottom (rectally).

Recommend to seek immediate medical help if her daughter, up to 12 months old, has a temperature of 39 °C or higher.

Discuss non-pharmacologic fever management strategies:

- Remove excess clothing or blanket
- The room should be comfortable, not too hot or cool
- A lukewarm bath or sponge bath may help

- Avoid cold baths, ice, or alcohol rubs. They initially cool the skin, but often worsen the condition by raising the core body temperature
- Circulating fans

Summarize and assess patient's understanding

Interactive case #36: Proper Use of Inhaler
Pharmacist – Standardized Patient Interaction

Your (Candidate) instructions

Case description:

Mr. Lee has been a long-time smoker. After few months of recurrent cough, he has been diagnosed with congestive obstructive pulmonary disease (COPD). He is coming to see you with a new prescription for Atroven HFA. He is looking forward learning from the pharmacist how to use his puffer properly. Assist the patient as you would in practice.

This station must be completed in 7 minutes

Station materials and references:

Patient profile
Compendium of Products for Minor Ailments
Atroven HFA

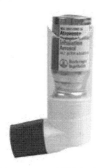

Atrovent HFA ©Boehringer Ingelheim Inc.

Patient profile

Patient Name: Matt Lee
Gender: Male
Age: 67 years old
Allergies: None
Medical History: Peptic ulcer, glaucoma
Current medications (Rx & nRx): Losec 20 mg daily, dorzolamide 1 drop Q8, 1 daily multivitamin, Tylenol prn for occasional back pain
New prescription: Atroven HFA 4 puffs Q8 daily
Social/lifestyle: Retired, lives alone with family support, stopped smoking 3 years ago, no alcohol intake, enjoys swimming – 3 times weekly

Standardized patient introductions and questions

<u>Case description:</u>

Mr. Lee has been a long-time smoker. After few months of recurrent cough, he has been diagnosed with congestive obstructive pulmonary disease (COPD). He is coming to see the pharmacist with a new prescription for Atroven HFA. He is looking forward learning from the pharmacist how to use his puffer properly.

Patient profile

Patient Name: Matt Lee
Gender: Male
Age: 67 years old
Allergies: None
Medical History: Peptic ulcer, glaucoma
Current medications (Rx & nRx): Losec 20 mg daily, dorzolamide 1 drop Q8, 1 daily multivitamin, Tylenol prn for occasional back pain
New prescription: Atroven HFA 4 puffs Q8 daily
Social/lifestyle: Retired, lives alone with family support, stopped smoking 3 years ago, no alcohol intake, enjoys swimming – 3 times weekly

If asked, Mr. Lee will provide the following additional information:

His glaucoma and ulcer are well controlled with medication

"Hi, I just got this new prescription from my physician. It is my first time taking this medication and I am not sure how to use it properly. I am also wondering if I can use it if I have a sudden attack"

If not addressed by the candidate after 4 minutes, the standardized patient will ask the following questions:

"Can I use it if I have a sudden attack?"

"What should I do if I forget my medication?"

CASE REVIEW FORM

Write notes, answers, interview and counselling to show how you would solve this case

Solution – Interactive Case #36

<u>Primary goals</u>:

- Educate the patient on how to use the inhaler
- Recommend monitoring the patient's glaucoma

The candidate is expected to:
Discuss the drug schedule with the patient. 4 puffs every 8 hours.
Explain how to use the Metered Dose Inhaler (MDI):
- Atroven HFA is a solution aerosol that does not require shaking
- Remove the cap
- Prime with 2 test sprays before first use. If the inhaler has not been used for more than 3 days, prime again by releasing 2 test sprays into the air away from the face. Each inhaler provides 200 inhalations.
- Breathe out, away from your inhaler
- Bring the inhaler to your mouth. Place it in your mouth between your teeth and close your mouth around it.
- Start to breathe in slowly. Press the top of you inhaler once and keep breathing in slowly until you have taken a full breath.
- Remove the inhaler from your mouth, and hold your breath for about 10 seconds, then breathe out.
- Wait 30s to 1 min before another puff. Repeat steps 3 to 6.
- Store the MDI at room temperature. If it gets cold, warm it using only your hands. When using a new MDI, write the start date on the canister. Check the expiry date on the MDI before use.
- Avoid contact with eyes to help minimize adverse effect on eye such as worsening of glaucoma. Recommend regular eye monitoring because the patient has glaucoma and to seek medical help immediately if vision changes
- Do not exceed 12 inhalations in 24 hours.

If you miss a dose, use it as soon as you remember it. If it is almost time for the next dose, skip the missed dose and carry on with regular schedule. Do not double a dose to make up for a missed one.

Discus common side effects: urinary retention, dry mouth, metallic taste (rinse mouth following drug administration)

Explain that Atroven HFA (Ipratropium) should not be used to treat sudden breathing problems where fast relief is needed. Fast acting medications (e.g., salbutamol, terbutaline) should be used for acute treatment. Refer the patient to his physician to determine if he needs such medication.
Discuss non-pharmacologic strategies:
- Avoid exposure to air pollution
- Physical activity helps improve symptoms

Assess patient understanding.

Interactive case #37: Insulin Pen
Pharmacist – Standardized Patient Interaction

Your (Candidate) instructions

Case description:

Ms. Smith has been diagnosed with type 2 Diabetes almost one year ago and has been using metformin. Unfortunately, her blood glucose level is still not well controlled. She is coming to see you with a new prescription for NovoRapid (Insulin Aspart). For added convenience and ease of injection an insulin pen has been prescribed. Ms. Smith is very eager to learn how to use properly her insulin pen. Please, provide your assistance.

This station must be completed in 7 minutes

Station materials and references: Patient profile
Compendium of Products for Minor Ailments
Novolin-Pen 4

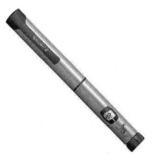

Novolin Pen 4 ©Novo Nordisk Inc.

Patient profile

Patient Name: Mary Smith
Gender: Female
Age: 53 years old
Allergies: None known
Medical History: Type 2 diabetes, hyperlipidemia
Current medications (Rx & nRx): Metformin 500 mg TID, fenofibrate 100 mg TID with meals
New prescription: NovoRapid Penfill 3ml 4 units before meals, Novolin-Pen 4
Social/lifestyle: Non-smoker, no alcohol use, physically active in average 4 times weekly

Standardized patient introductions and questions

Case description:

Ms. Smith has been diagnosed with type 2 Diabetes almost one year ago and has been using metformin. Unfortunately, her blood glucose level is still not well controlled. She is coming to see the pharmacist with a new prescription for NovoRapid (Insulin Aspart). For added convenience and ease of injection an insulin pen has been prescribed. Ms. Smith is very eager to learn how to use properly her insulin pen.

Patient profile

Patient Name: Mary Smith
Gender: Female
Age: 53 years old
Allergies: None known
Medical History: Type 2 diabetes, hyperlipidemia
Current medications (Rx & nRx): Metformin 500 mg TID, fenofibrate 100 mg TID with meals
New prescription: NovoRapid Penfill 3ml 4 units before meals, Novolin-Pen 4
Social/lifestyle: Non-smoker, no alcohol use, physically active in average 4 times weekly

"Hi, I just got this new prescription from my physician. It is my first time using insulin. My physician has recommended the pen. Could you show me how to use it? Should I stop using my other medication?"

If not addressed by the candidate after 4 minutes, the standardized patient will ask the following questions:

"When should I use my insulin?"

"Do I have to always keep the pen in the refrigerator?"

CASE REVIEW FORM

Write notes, answers, interview and counselling to show how you would solve this case

Solution – Interactive case #37

<u>Primary goal</u>:

Educate the patient

The candidate is expected to:

The candidate is expected to:

Advise injecting 4 units of insulin 5 to 10 minutes before or immediately after a meal.

Show how to use the insulin pen.

Explain that insulin aspart is fast acting and provides good blood sugar control after a meal. Do not inject if you are not planning to have a meal.

Explain that she can inject insulin aspart in her thighs, stomach, upper arms, or buttocks. Recommend rotating the injection site within the chosen area with each dose; try to avoid injecting the same site more often than once every 1 to 2 weeks. Warn that she may experience redness and irritation at the site of injection.

Advise to always check insulin aspart before injecting it. It should be clear and colorless (like water). Do not use if it is colored, cloudy, thickened, or contains solid particles, or if the expiration date on the bottle has passed.

Advise the patient to store unopened insulin aspart cartridges in the refrigerator but not to freeze them. Unopened refrigerated insulin aspart can be stored until the expiration date. Unrefrigerated pens can be used within 28 days. Avoid exposure to sunlight and high temperatures.

Explain that she should not stop using metformin unless her physician decides otherwise. Metformin and insulin work together to help control better her blood sugar. Advise periodic monitoring.
Advise the patient to seek medical help if she experiences any of the following symptoms:

- Rash and/or itching over the whole body
- Shortness of breath
- Wheezing
- Dizziness
- Blurred vision
- Fast heartbeat
- Sweating
- Weakness

Recall the importance of non-pharmacologic strategies including health diet, physical activity, self-monitoring and periodic reassessments. Assess patient understanding.

Interactive case #38: Oral Contraceptives
Pharmacist – Standardized Patient Interaction

Your (Candidate) instructions

Case description:

A young female is visiting your pharmacy with a prescription for oral contraceptive Min-Ovral28. She is very much concerned about confidentiality because her mother, who is not aware of her decision, is your regular patient. She is expecting to learn about the proper use of the contraceptive and how to deal with missed dose to avoid unwanted pregnancy. A friend told her that the medication will also help control her acne. Please, assist the patient as you would in practice.

This station must be completed in 7 minutes

Station materials and references:

Compendium of Therapeutic Choices (CTC)
No patient profile

Note: the standardized patient shows signs of anxiousness.

Standardized patient introductions and questions

Case description:

A young female is visiting the pharmacy with a prescription for oral contraceptive Min-Ovral 28. She is very much concerned about confidentiality because her mother, who is not aware of her decision, visits the pharmacy regularly. She is expecting to learn about the proper use of the contraceptive and how to deal with missed dose to avoid unwanted pregnancy. A friend told her that the medication will also help control her acne.

If asked, the patient will provide the following information:

Patient Name: Karen Singh
Gender: Female
Age: 16 years old
Allergies: None known
Medical History: None
Current medications (Rx & nRx): None
New prescription: Ovral28

She is not a smoker
Social/lifestyle: High school student, non-smoker, no alcohol intake, physically active – cheerleading, swimming and soccer
It is her first prescription for oral contraceptives
Until now, she has been sexually inactive

"Hi, I just got this new prescription from my physician. It is my first time taking this medication and I have many questions. First of all could you keep it between us? I would like to know how to take the medication and what to expect? A friend told me that it will help my acne? Is it true? What should I do if I miss a pill?"

Note: the standardized patient shows signs of anxiousness.

If not addressed by the candidate after 4 minutes, the standardized patient must ask the following questions:

"What if I miss a pill?"

"When should I start using it?

CASE REVIEW FORM

Write notes, answers, interview and counselling to show how you would solve this case

Solution – Interactive Case #38

Primary goal:

Educate the patient on the use of oral contraceptives

The candidate is expected to:

Ensure confidentiality.

Warn that the use of oral contraceptives does not protect against sexually transmitted diseases such as HIV infection. Recommend the use of latex condoms for protection against sexually transmitted diseases (STDs).

Confirm that the patient is not a smoker; smoking increases the risk of cardiovascular adverse effects.

Explain that Ovral is very effective if used as prescribed; the failure rate is lower than 0.1%. Therefore, it is important to take the pills according to schedule.

Confirm that oral contraceptives do improve acne
Discuss the medication schedule: take 1 "active" pill daily for 21 days, then take 1 "reminder or inactive" pill daily for 7 days, and then begin the next pack. The pills should be taken approximately the same time every day, preferably after the evening meal or at bedtime. The pills can be taken with or without food. She should start taking her pills on Day 1 or Day 5 of her period.

Recommend using a second method of birth control (e.g., abstinence, latex condoms and spermicidal foam or gel) for the first 7 days of the first cycle of pill use.

Explain that she may experience unexpected bleeding and spotting, especially at the beginning of pill use. It is important to continue taking the pills every day even if she is spotting or bleeding, or has an upset stomach. Do not stop taking oral contraceptives without talking to her physician.

Explain that if she vomits a dose of the medication within 4 hours of taking it, the medication may not be effective. She must assume it is a missed dose then follow the instructions for a missed dose.

Discuss that the medication has the following common side effects: breakthrough bleeding/spotting, amenorrhea, nausea/vomiting, chloasma, breast tenderness, mood changes and headaches. Oral contraceptives will also help regulate her menstrual cycle and decrease menstrual flow.

Explain how to manage a missed pill:

- If you miss one pill, take it as soon as you remember, and take the next pill at the usual time. This means that it is likely that you take 2 pills in one day.
- If you miss 2 pills in a row during the first 2 weeks of your cycle, take 2 pills on the day you remember and 2 pills the next day. Then take one pill a day until you finish the pack. Use a second method of birth control if you have sex in the 7 days after you missed the pills.
- If you miss 2 pills in a row during the third week of your cycle or 3 or more pills at any time during your cycle, safely dispose of the rest of the pill pack and start a new pack that same day. Use another method of birth control if you have sex in the 7 days after you missed the pills. You may miss your period this month. If you miss 2 periods in a row, call your physician.

Assess patient understanding

Interactive case #39: Treatment of H. Pylori Infection
Pharmacist – Standardized Patient Interaction

Your (Candidate) instructions

Case description:

Mrs. Paul has been dealing with recurrent peptic ulcer for the past few months. She has been just diagnosed with H. Pylori infection and is coming to see you with a prescription for Hp-PAC. Please, provide your assistance.

This station must be completed in 7 minutes

Station materials and references:

Patient profile
Compendium of Products for Minor Ailments
Rx Files chart

Patient profile

Patient Name: Helen Paul
Gender: Female
Age: 45 years old
Allergies: Penicillin allergy
Medical History: Peptic ulcer
Current medications (Rx & nRx): Pepto Bismol prn
New prescription: Hp-PAC BID for 7 days
Social/lifestyle: Accountant, non-smoker, moderate alcohol intake – 3 to 5 drinks weekly

Standardized patient introductions and questions

Case description:

Mrs. Paul has been dealing with recurrent peptic ulcer for the past few months. She has been just diagnosed with H. Pylori infection and is coming to see you with a prescription for Hp-PAC.

Patient profile

Patient Name: Helen Paul
Gender: Female
Age: 45 years old
Allergies: Penicillin allergy
Medical History: Peptic ulcer
Current medications (Rx & nRx): None
New prescription: Hp-PAC BID for 7 days
Social/lifestyle: Accountant, non-smoker, moderate alcohol intake – 3 to 5 drinks weekly

"Hi, I just got this new prescription from my physician for my ulcer. Could you explain how I should use it and for how long? Could you also tell me what to expect?"

If asked, provide the following additional information:

She was previously treatment for ulcer but her symptoms kept coming back.

If not addressed by the candidate after 4 minutes, the standardized patient will ask the following questions:

"What should I expect while taking this medication?"

"Should I stop using Pepto Bismol completely?"

CASE REVIEW FORM

Write notes, answers, interview and counselling to show how you would solve this case

Solution – Interactive Case #39

Primary goals:

- Determine that Hp-PAC is contraindicated in patients with penicillin allergy because it contains amoxicillin. Hp-PAC is a first line triple therapy for the eradication of H. Pylori and contains lansoprazole 30mg po BID, amoxicillin 1000mg po BID and clarithromycin 500mg po BID. Avoid Losec 1-2-3 A which contains also amoxicillin: omeprazole 20mg po BID, amoxicillin 1000mg po BID, clarithromycin 500mg po BID

- Switch the patient to Losec 1-2-3 M which is also a first line triple therapy. Losec 1-2-3 M contains omeprazole 20mg po BID, metronidazole 500mg po BID and clarithromycin 250mg po BID.

The candidate is expected to:

Explain that based on her history of penicillin allergy Hp-PAC is contraindicated because it contains a penicillin-like product.

Reassure the patient that her physician will be contacted to prescribe another effective medication (Losec 1-2-3 M) that suits her profile.

Advise not to drink alcohol during the duration of treatment to prevent the likelihood of flushing, fast heart rate, confusion, nausea, vomiting and syncope (metronidazole related disulfiram reaction).

Discuss common side effects: diarrhea and taste disturbances

Explain the drug schedule: twice a day for 7 days

Recommend using Pepto Bismol to manage occasional symptoms during treatment. Short term use of acid suppression is recommended until complete eradication of H. Pylori is achieved.

Summarize and assess patient understanding

Interactive case #40: Application of Nasal Spray
Pharmacist – Standardized Patient Interaction

Your (Candidate) instructions

Case description:

A young male patient is coming to see you regarding the proper use of a nonprescription nasal spray. He has a cold and has been dealing with nasal congestion for two days. He would like also to know how many sprays will be needed and for how long he can use it.
Please, provide your assistance.

This station must be completed in 7 minutes

Station materials and references:
Compendium of Products for Minor Ailments
No patient's profile
Afrin PumpMist

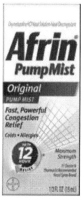

Afrin Pump Mist ©Bayer Inc.

Standardized patient introductions and questions

Case description:

A young male patient is coming to see the pharmacist regarding the proper use of a nonprescription nasal spray. He has a cold and has been dealing with nasal congestion for two days. He would like also to know how many sprays will be needed and for how long he can use it.

There is no patient's profile in this station. If asked, provide the following information:

Patient Name: Sam Michael
Age: 20 years old
Allergies: None
Medical History: None
Current medications (Rx & nRx): None
Social/lifestyle: College student, non-smoker, no alcohol intake, plays volleyball at least 3 times a week

He has a cold and has been dealing with nasal congestion for 2 days.

"Hi, I just got this nasal spray. I have been dealing with stuffy nose for two days, I have a cold. Could you show me how to use it properly? How many sprays do I need?"

If not addressed by the candidate after 4 minutes, the standardized patient will ask:

"How many sprays do I need?"

"For how long can I use it?"

CASE REVIEW FORM

Write notes, answers, interview and counselling to show how you would solve this case

Solution – Interactive case #40

<u>Primary goal</u>:

Demonstration of the use of Afrin PumpMist
Recommend not to use the spray for more than 3 days to avoid rebound congestion

The candidate is expected to:

Demonstrate and explain the proper use of Afrin PumpMist:

- Shake well before use
- Before first use, remove the cap and prime the pump by depressing firmly several times
- To spray, do not tilt the head. Simply insert the nozzle in the nostril and depress firmly, then sniff deeply.
- Wipe clean the nozzle

2 to 3 sprays in each nostril not more often than 10 to 12 hours; do not exceed 2 doses in 24 hours.
Side effects include stinging, burning, sneezing or increased nasal discharge
Do not use more than 3 days to prevent rebound congestion (worsening of congestion)

Discuss non-pharmacologic strategies:

- Use gentle saline nasal sprays.
- Increase the humidity in the air with a vaporizer or humidifier.
- Drink extra fluids. Hot tea, broth, or chicken soup

Summarize and assess patient understanding

Interactive case #41: Acne Treatment
Pharmacist – Standardized Patient Interaction

Your (Candidate) instructions

Case description:

Ms. Young has been using Reversa 15% for the past 6 weeks for the treatment of acne. Unfortunately her condition has not improved significantly. One of her friends who used Accutane recently told her that it is very effective. She is now considering using Accutane. She would like to have your opinion before finalizing her decision. Please, provide your assistance.

This station must be completed in 7 minutes

Station materials and references:

Patient profile
Drugs in Pregnancy and Lactation
Compendium of Therapeutic Choices (CTC)

Patient profile

Patient Name: Pam Young
Gender: Female
Age: 21 years old
Allergies: None known
Medical History: None
Current medications (Rx & nRx): Centrum Materna 1 tablet daily
Social/lifestyle: Graduate student, non-smoker, no alcohol intake

Standardized patient introductions and questions

Case description:

Ms. Young has been using Reversa 15% for the past 6 weeks for the treatment of acne. Unfortunately her condition has not improved significantly. One of her friends who used Accutane recently told her that it is very effective. She is now considering using Accutane. She would like to have the pharmacist's opinion before finalizing her decision.

Patient profile

Patient Name: Pam Young
Gender: Female
Age: 21 years old
Allergies: None known
Medical History: None
Current medications (Rx & nRx): Centrum Materna 1 tablet daily
Social/lifestyle: Graduate student, non-smoker, no alcohol intake

"Hi, I am thinking about using Accutane for my acne. One of my friends is really happy using it, it works. I would like to have your advice. It will be my first time using it."

If asked, she will provide the following additional information:

I have been using Reversa15% for the past 6 weeks. My acne has not improved significantly.

I am about 2 months pregnant.

If not addressed by the candidate after 4 minutes, the patient will ask:

"What else do you suggest?"

CASE REVIEW FORM

Write notes, answers, interview and counselling to show how you would solve this case

Solution – Interactive Case #41

Primary goals:

- Determine that the patient is pregnant
- Explain that Accutane is contraindicated during pregnancy

The candidate is expected to:

To confirm that Ms. Young is pregnant by asking questions. Accutane is contraindicated during pregnancy. Her profile shows daily use of Centrum Materna

Explain that Accutane (Isotretinoin) is contraindicated during pregnancy. Isotretinoin is a proven teratogenic (capable of causing malformations in the fetus) agent.

Explain that Reversa 15% (15% glycolic acid) is also effective. Recommend using it for a longer period.

Summarize and assess patient understanding

Interactive case #42: Garlic Supplement
Pharmacist – Standardized Patient Interaction

Your (Candidate) instructions

Case description:

Mr. Ryan is visiting the pharmacy located in a Shopping Mall to seek your advice regarding garlic supplements. He learned from few friends that garlic has several health benefits. He is wondering if he should start using it for his heart problems. Mr. Ryan is already taking two heart medications. Please, provide your assistance.

This station must be completed in 7 minutes

Station materials and references:

Natural Medicines Comprehensive Database

Standardized patient introductions and questions

Case description:

Mr. Ryan is visiting the pharmacy located in a Shopping Mall to seek the pharmacist's advice regarding garlic supplement. He learned from few friends that garlic has several health benefits. He is wondering if he should start using it for his heart problems. Mr. Ryan is already taking two heart medications.

"Hi, I would like to have your advice regarding garlic supplements. Do you think I should start using it for my heart problems? At least two of my friends are using it. I am thinking about adding it to my shopping list"

There is no patient profile in this station. If asked, the patient will provide the following information:

He is 59 years old.

At least two of his friends are taking garlic supplements.

It is his first time visiting the pharmacy. He just decided to stop by because the location is convenient. His regular pharmacy is in a different location.

He has been using heart medications for 3 years. He can't tell exactly what kind of heart medications he is taking.

CASE REVIEW FORM

Write notes, answers, interview and counselling to show how you would solve this case

Solution – Interactive Case #42

Primary goals:

- Provide an overview of garlic supplements and their potential health benefits
- Refer the client to his pharmacist or physician to determine if he can safely use garlic supplements.

The candidate is expected to some extent to:

Explain that garlic has beneficial effects on high blood pressure, high cholesterol, coronary heart disease, heart attack, and hardening of the arteries (atherosclerosis). It is also used in the prevention of colon cancer, rectal cancer, stomach cancer, breast cancer, prostate cancer, and lung cancer.

Discuss that choosing the right supplement is very important. There is a lot of variation among garlic supplements. The amount of allicin, the active ingredient and the source of garlic's distinctive odor, depends on the method of preparation. Allicin is unstable, and aging garlic to make it odorless reduces the amount of allicin resulting in the reduction of effectiveness.

Explain that in general garlic is safe in most people. Garlic can cause bad breath, a burning sensation in the mouth or stomach, heartburn, gas, nausea, vomiting, body odor, and diarrhea. These side effects are often worse with raw garlic.

Warn that garlic interacts with many medications such as:

Isoniazid (reduction of absorption and effectiveness)
Antiviral medications (increased metabolism of Non-Nucleoside Reverse Transcriptase Inhibitors and reduction of effectiveness)

Cytochrome P450 2E1 (CYP2E1) substrates including acetaminophen, chlorzoxazone, ethanol and theophylline. (Increased bioavailability)

Cytochrome P450 3A4 (CYP3A4) substrates including certain heart medications called calcium channel blockers (diltiazem, nicardipine, verapamil), cancer drugs (etoposide, paclitaxel, vinblastine, vincristine, vindesine), antifungal drugs (ketoconazole, itraconazole), glucocorticoids, alfentanil, cisapride, fentanyl, lidocaine, losartan, midazolam , and others. (Reduction of effectiveness)

Anticoagulant / Antiplatelet drugs including aspirin, clopidogrel, diclofenac, ibuprofen, naproxen, dalteparin, enoxaparin, heparin, warfarin, and others. (Increased anticoagulant effect)

Refer the client to his pharmacist or physician to determine if he can safely use garlic supplements.

Summarize and assess patient understanding.

Interactive case #43: Phenobarbital Counselling
Pharmacist – Standardized Patient Interaction

Your (Candidate) instructions

Case description:

Mrs. Thomas has been diagnosed recently with partial seizures. She is coming to see you with a new prescription for phenobarbital. She would like to know how to use the medication and what to expect. Please, provide your assistance.

This station must be completed in 7 minutes

Station materials and references:

Patient profile
Drugs in Pregnancy and Lactation

Patient profile

Patient Name: Jessie Thomas
Gender: Female
Age: 31 years old
Allergies: None known
Medical History: None
Current medications (Rx & nRx): Centrum Materna 1 tablet daily
Social/lifestyle: Non-smoker, no alcohol intake
New prescription: Phenobarbital 90 mg daily hs for 4 weeks

Standardized patient introductions and questions

<u>Case description</u>:

Mrs. Thomas has been diagnosed recently with partial seizures. She is coming to see the pharmacist with a new prescription for phenobarbital. She would like to know how to use the medication and what to expect.

Patient profile

Patient Name: Jessie Thomas
Gender: Female
Age: 31 years old
Allergies: None known
Medical History: None
Current medications (Rx & nRx): Centrum Materna 1 tablet daily
Social/lifestyle: Non-smoker, no alcohol intake
New prescription: Phenobarbital 90 mg daily hs for 4 weeks

"Hi, I just got this new prescription from my physician. It's my first time taking this medication. Could you tell me how to take it and what to expect?"

If asked, the standardized patient will provide the following additional information:

She had a son 3 months ago.

She is breastfeeding and plan to continue until her baby is at least one year old.

She doesn't work; she takes care of her son.

CASE REVIEW FORM

Write notes, answers, interview and counselling to show how you would solve this case

Solution – Interactive Case #43

<u>Primary goals</u>:

- Determine that Mrs. Thomas is breastfeeding
- Explain that phenobarbital is excreted in large amounts in breast milk and could adversely affect her baby

Patient profile

Patient Name: Jessie Thomas
Gender: Female
Age: 31 years old
Allergies: None known
Medical History: None
Current medications (Rx & nRx): Centrum Materna 1 tablet daily
Social/lifestyle: Non-smoker, no alcohol intake
New prescription: Phenobarbital 90 mg daily hs for 4 weeks

The candidate is expected to:

Determine that Mrs. Thomas is breastfeeding

Explain that Phenobarbital is excreted in large amounts in breast milk and could adversely affect her baby.

Reassure the patient that her physician will be called to prescribe another medication. Phenobarbital is not a first choice monotherapy. First choice montherapy for partial seizures are: carbamazepine, lamotrigine and phenytoin.

Discuss non-pharmacologic options such as avoidance of sleep deprivation, minimum intake of alcohol. Cocaine and amphetamines must be forbidden due to their proconvulsant properties. Some patient could also benefit from support groups.

Discuss safety precautions:

- To reduce the incidence of burns avoid smoking and encourage the use of microwave
- Showers are preferred over bathes to reduce the risk of drowning
- Recommend not to bath the baby without supervision
- Recommend not to use change tables for clothing or changing the baby
- Avoid driving without supervision

Recommend folic acid supplementation; 5 mg/day is recommended for women of child bearing potential to reduce the teratogenic effects of anticonvulsants.

Summarize and assess patient understanding.

Interactive case #44: Sunscreen Counselling
Pharmacist – Standardized Client Interaction

Your (Candidate) instructions

Case description:

A client is seeking your assistance to select a sunscreen for her two grandchildren. Mrs. Kim is preparing for a vacation in sunny Cancun, Mexico. As expected, she is concerned about potential damaging effects of sun exposure. She would like also to learn how to use the sunscreen properly. Please, provide your assistance.

This station must be completed in 7 minutes

Station materials and references:

Compendium of Products for Minor Ailments
There is no patient profile

Standardized client introductions and questions

Case description:

A client is seeking the pharmacist's assistance to select a sunscreen for her two grandchildren. Mrs. Kim is preparing for a vacation in sunny Cancun, Mexico. As expected, she is concerned about potential damaging effects of sun exposure. She would like also to learn how to use the sunscreen properly.

"Hi, we are leaving next week for a vacation in Cancun, Mexico. I am wondering if you can help me select a good sunscreen for my two grandchildren. Could you also tell me how to use it properly?"

If asked, the standardized client will provide the following additional information:

Her grandchildren are 4 months and 3 years old

If not addressed by the candidate after 4 minutes, the standardized client will ask the following questions:

"Can I use the same sunscreen for both children?"

"Do I need to apply it and wait for a while before heading outside?"

CASE REVIEW FORM

Write notes, answers, interview and counselling to show how you would solve this case

Solution – Interactive Case #44

Primary goals:

- Interview the client to determine the age of the children.
- Recommend a physical sunscreen which is suitable for people of all ages including infants.

The candidate is expected to:

Interview the client to determine the age of the children.

Recommend and explain that physical sunscreens protect against UVA and UVB and contain titanium oxide, zinc oxide, kaolin, talc (magnesium silicate), ferric chloride or melanin. They provide immediate protection following application. Recommend at least SPF 30.

Explain that chemical sunscreens are used in children older than 6 months and should be applied 15 to 60 minutes before sun exposure. They contain UVA and UVB absorbers such as padimate O, homosalate, oxybenzone, camphor, Parsol …

Explain that waterproof sunscreens retain their efficacy for 80 minutes following swimming; water-resistant sunscreens remain active for 40 minutes following swimming. Reapply after swimming for regular sunscreens.

Reapplying the sunscreen 15 to 30 minutes after sun exposure enhances protection but does not extend the period of protection.

Explain that a sunscreen does not provide complete protection. Sunscreens should be adjunctive rather than primary means of protection.

Discuss the following non-pharmacologic strategies:

- Avoid outdoor activities at peak UV period between 10:00 am and 4:00 pm
- Ideally outdoor activities should be in the shade. Umbrellas reduce UV radiation by up to 70%.
- Wear protective clothing such as pants, long-sleeved shirts, wide-brimmed hats….

Explain how to treat minor sunburns:

- Apply cool or wet compresses for 20 minutes four to six times
- Apply moisturizers to prevent dryness and peeling
- Drink lot of fluids
- After sunburn, the affected area should not be exposed to sun for at least a week.

Summarize and assess client understanding.

Interactive case #45: St. John's Wort
Pharmacist – Standardized Patient Interaction

Your (Candidate) instructions

Case description:

Mrs. Smith is visiting the pharmacy located in a Shopping Mall to seek your advice regarding St. John's wort. She learned from the internet that her occasional feelings of sadness can be managed with St. John's wort. She is wondering if she should start using it. Mrs. Smith is already taking one medication for anxiety and another one for her irregular heart rhythms. Please, provide your assistance.

This station must be completed in 7 minutes

Station materials and references:

Natural Medicines Comprehensive Database

Standardized patient introductions and questions

Case description:

Mrs. Smith is visiting the pharmacy located in a Shopping Mall to seek the pharmacist's advice regarding St. John's wort. She learned from the internet that her occasional feelings of sadness can be managed with St. John's wort. She is wondering if she should start using it. Mrs. Smith is already taking one medication for anxiety and another one for her irregular heart rhythms.

"Hi, I would like to have your advice regarding St. John's wort. I learned on the internet that it could be good for my occasional sadness. Do you think I should start using it? I am ready to add it to my shopping list"

There is no patient profile in this station. If requested, the standardized client will provide the following information:

She is 53 years old

It is her first time visiting the pharmacy. She just decided to stop by because the location is convenient. Her regular pharmacy is in a different location.

She doesn't know exactly what the two medications she is taking are. She started using both 3 months ago.

CASE REVIEW FORM

Write notes, answers, interview and counselling to show how you would solve this case

Solution – Interactive case #45

Primary goals:

- Provide an overview of the use of St. John's wort
- Refer the client to her physician to evaluate the effectiveness of her anxiety medication and to determine if she is a good candidate for St. John's wort.

The candidate is expected to some extent to:

Explain that St. John's wort is an herb. Medicines are made using its flowers and leaves. St. John's wort is primarily used for depression based on some strong scientific evidence. It also used to treat anxiety, tiredness, loss of appetite and trouble sleeping disorders. Other uses include heart palpitations, symptoms of menopause (mood), attention deficit-hyperactivity disorder (ADHD), obsessive-compulsive disorder (OCD), and seasonal affective disorder (SAD).

Explain that St. John's wort is in general safe for most people. It can cause some side effects such as trouble sleeping, vivid dreams, restlessness, anxiety, irritability, stomach upset, fatigue, dry mouth, dizziness, headache, skin rash, diarrhea, and tingling.

Warn that St, John's wort interacts with many medications:

Cytochrome P450 2C19 (CYP2C19) substrates (decreased effectiveness): amitriptyline, citalopram, diazepam, lansoprazole, omeprazole, phenytoin, warfarin, and many others.

Cytochrome P450 3A4 (CYP3A4) substrates (decreased effectiveness): lovastatin, ketoconazole, itraconazole, fexofenadine, triazolam, and many others.

Antidepressant drugs (synergistic effect): fluoxetine, paroxetine, sertraline, amitriptyline, clomipramine, imipramine, and others.

Medications for HIV/AIDS medications (reduced effectiveness)

Photosensitizing drugs (increased sunlight sensitivity): amitriptyline, Ciprofloxacin, norfloxacin, lomefloxacin, ofloxacin, levofloxacin, sparfloxacin, gatifloxacin, moxifloxacin, trimethoprim/sulfamethoxazole and others.

Refer the client to her physician to evaluate the effectiveness of her anxiety medication and to determine if she is a good candidate for St. John's wort.

Summarize and assess patient understanding

Interactive case #46: Analgesic
Pharmacist – Standardized Patient Interaction

Your (Candidate) instructions

Case description:

Mrs. John is 32 weeks pregnant. She is visiting the pharmacy to purchase a nonprescription analgesic for her back pain. Mrs. John is hesitant because she is aware that many medications should be avoided during pregnancy. She decided wisely to seek your assistance. Please, help Mrs. John as you would in practice.

This station must be completed in 7 minutes

Station materials and references:

Patient profile
Drugs in Pregnancy and Lactation
Advil and Tylenol

Patient profile

Patient Name: Amanda John
Gender: Female
Age: 25 years old
Allergies: None known
Medical History: None
Current medications (Rx & nRx): Centrum Materna 1 tablet daily
Social/lifestyle: Teacher, non-smoker, no alcohol intake

Standardized patient introductions and questions

Case description:

Mrs. John is 32 weeks pregnant. She is visiting the pharmacy to purchase a nonprescription analgesic for her back pain. Mrs. John is hesitant because she is aware that many medications should be avoided during pregnancy. She decided wisely to seek the pharmacist's assistance.

Patient profile

Patient Name: Amanda John
Gender: Female
Age: 25 years old
Allergies: None known
Medical History: None
Current medications (Rx & nRx): Centrum Materna 1 tablet daily
Social/lifestyle: Teacher, non-smoker, no alcohol intake

"Hi, I have been suffering from back pain since yesterday. Could you help me select a medication for pain? Which of these two products will be best for me?"

Two nonprescription pain medications are available in the station.

If asked, she will provide the following additional information:

She is 32 weeks pregnant.

CASE REVIEW FORM

Write notes, answers, interview and counselling to show how you would solve this case

Solution – Interactive Case #46

<u>Primary goal</u>:

Recommend Tylenol; NSAIDs should be avoided especially during the third trimester of pregnancy due to increased risk of maternal and fetal bleeding

The candidate is expected to:

Explain that back pain is common during pregnancy due to among others weight gain. Recommend Tylenol

Explain that NSAIDs should be avoided especially during the third trimester of pregnancy due to increased risk of maternal and fetal bleeding.

Discuss the following non-pharmacologic strategies.

Practice good posture:

- Stand up straight and tall.
- Hold your chest high.
- Keep your shoulders back and relaxed.
- Don't lock your knees.

Sitting with care is also important. Choose a chair that supports your back, or place a small pillow behind your lower back. Keep your upper back and neck comfortably straight. Consider elevating your feet on a low stool.

Wear low-heeled shoes with good support. Wear maternity pants with a low, supportive waistband. A maternity support belt could also help.

Sleep on your side, not your back. Keep one or both knees bent. It might also help to place one pillow between your knees and another under your abdomen, or use a full-length body pillow.

Use a heating pad to apply heat to your back, or alternate ice packs with heat. Rubbing your back could also help.

Regular physical activity can keep your back strong and could relieve back pain during pregnancy. Try gentle activities such as walking or swimming.

Warn that a low, dull backache might be a sign of preterm labor. Severe back pain or back pain coupled with vaginal bleeding or discharge could indicate a problem that needs immediate attention.
Recommend that she talks to her physician if her back pain persists

Summarize and assess patient understanding.

Interactive case #47: Osteoporosis
Pharmacist – Standardized Patient Interaction

Your (Candidate) instructions

Case description:

Mrs Summer is a postmenopausal woman who has been just diagnosed with osteoporosis. She is already taking daily supplements of calcium and vitamin D. Her physician has prescribed once weekly 70 mg alendronate (Foxamax) for treatment. She is expecting to learn from the pharmacist how to take the medication and what to expect. She is also concerned about storage conditions. Please, provide your assistance.

This station must be completed in 7 minutes

Station materials and references:

Patient profile
Compendium of Pharmaceuticals and Specialties (CPS)
Compendium of Products for Minor Ailments

Patient profile

Patient Name: Lynn Summer
Gender: Female
Age: 58 years old
Allergies: Seasonal allergies
Medical History: Hyperlypidemia, shingles
Current medications (Rx & nRx): Fenofibrate 160mg daily, amitriptyline 10 mg tab qhs – started 5 weeks ago, one multivitamin daily, calcium 800 mg daily, vitamin D 400 IU, one omega-3 capsule
New prescription: Foxamax 70 mg once weekly
Social/lifestyle: Non-smoker, no alcohol use, physically active – daily yoga classes

Standardized patient introductions and questions

Case description:

Mrs Summer is a postmenopausal woman who has been just diagnosed with osteoporosis. She is already taking daily supplements of calcium and vitamin D. Her physician has prescribed once weekly 70 mg alendronate (Foxamax) for treatment. She is expecting to learn from the pharmacist how to take the medication and what to expect. She is also concerned about storage conditions.

Patient profile

Patient Name: Lynn Summer
Gender: Female
Age: 58 years old
Allergies: Seasonal allergies
Medical History: Hyperlypidemia, shingles
Current medications (Rx & nRx): Fenofibrate 160 mg daily, amitriptyline 10 mg tab qhs – started 5 weeks ago, one multivitamin daily, calcium 800 mg daily, vitamin D 400 IU, one omega-3 capsule
New prescription: Foxamax 70 mg once weekly
Social/lifestyle: Non-smoker, no alcohol use, physically active – daily yoga classes

"Hi, I just got this new prescription from my physician. Could you explain how I should use it? Could you also tell me how to store it?"

If not addressed by the candidate, after 4 minutes, the standardized patient will ask the following questions:

"Can I take my other medications with this one?"

"What should I do if I miss a dose?"

"Can I keep the bottle on my desk?"

"What should I expect while taking this medication"

CASE REVIEW FORM

Write notes, answers, interview and counselling to show how you would solve this case

Solution – Interactive Case #47

Primary goal:

Patient education
The candidate is expected to:

Explain the medication schedule: Once a week

The candidate is expected to discuss:

Fosamax is not a hormone
Fosamax is used to treat and prevent osteoporosis
Improvement in bone density may be observed as early as 3 months after starting Fosamax

How to take once weekly Fosamax:
- Choose the day of the week that best fits your schedule.
- Take 1 dose of FOSAMAX every week on your chosen day after you get up for the day and before taking your first food, drink, or other medication – Take on empty stomach only
- Take FOSAMAX while you are sitting or standing.
- Take your FOSAMAX with plain water only
- Swallow one tablet with a full glass (6-8 oz) of plain water
- Do not chew or suck on a tablet of Fosamax

Do not take Fosamax with:
Mineral water
Coffee or tea
Juice

After taking your Fosamax, wait at least 30 minutes:
- Before you lie down. You may sit, stand or walk, and do normal activities.
- Before you take your first food or drink except for plain water.
- Before you take other medications, including antacids, calcium, and other supplements and vitamins.

If you miss a dose:
- Take only 1 dose of Fosamax on the morning after you remember
- Do not take 2 doses on the same day
- Then continue your usual schedule of 1 dose once a week on your chosen day

The most common side effect is abdominal pain. Less common side effects are nausea, vomiting, a full or bloated feeling in the stomach, constipation, diarrhea, black or bloody stools, gas, eye pain, rash that may be made worse by sunlight, hair loss, headache, dizziness, a changed sense of taste, joint swelling or swelling in the hands or legs, and bone, muscle, or joint pain.

Mouth sores (ulcers) may occur if the Fosamax tablet is chewed or dissolved in the mouth.

You may get flu-like symptoms, typically at the start of treatment with Fosamax.

You may get allergic reactions, such as hives or, in rare cases, swelling of your face, lips, tongue, or throat.

Fosamax may cause jaw-bone problems including infection, and delayed healing after teeth are pulled.

Store at room temperature

Recommend increasing her intake of calcium to 1200 mg daily and vitamin D to 800 IU

Discuss the importance of high impact physical activity such as walking and jogging

Summarize and assess patient understanding

Interactive Case #48
Pharmacist – Standardized Physician Interaction

Your (Candidate) instructions:

Case description:

You are a pharmacist in a community pharmacy. Dr. Kim calls from a drop-in clinic requesting some information regarding Benzaclin before prescribing it to his patient for the treatment of recurrent acne. The patient, Marlene Roberts has tried numerous acne over-the-counter products for the past 2 years without noticeable improvement. Dr. Kim would like to learn about precautions related to Benzaclin therapy. You are expected to help the physician make a safe prescribing decision. Refer to the physician's introduction and questions, **below**, to fully understand his expectations.

This station must be completed in 7 minutes

Station materials and references:
Compendium of Pharmaceuticals and Specialties (CPS)
Compendium of Therapeutic Choices (CTC)

Patient profile

Name: Marlene Roberts
Gender: Female
Age: 16 years old
Medical History: Recurrent acne
Allergies: None
Current Medications (Rx & nRx): OTC benzoyl peroxide
Social/lifestyle: Soccer player since age 9; plays the piano

Standardized physician introductions and questions

"Hi, I am Dr. Kim. I would like to clarify any precautions regarding Benzaclin before prescribing it to my patient for the treatment of recurrent acne. She has tried numerous OTC topical products without success. Are you aware of any precautions related to Benzaclin?"

If the candidate does not identify any precautions, then the standardized physician will add:

"So, it means Benzaclin is prescribed without concerns."

Other questions:

"What are the active ingredients in Benzaclin?"

If the candidate successfully identifies clindamycin **and** benzoyl peroxide, then the standardized physician will add:

"I know that an antibiotic alone could be effective in the treatment of acne. Why is benzoyl peroxide included?"

CASE REVIEW FORM

Write notes, answers, interview and counselling to show how you would solve this case

Solution – Interactive Case #48

<u>Primary goals</u>:

- Identify the precautions related to the use of Benzaclin
- List the active ingredients in Benzaclin
- Explain the addition of benzoyl peroxide

You are expected to provide the following information to Dr. Kim:

One of the active ingredients in Benzaclin, clindamycin, is known to induce antibiotic associated diarrhea. Therefore, Benzaclin should not be administered to patients with history of:
- Antibiotic-associated colitis
- Crohn's disease, ulcerative colitis, or inflammation of the small intestine

Benzaclin should also be avoided in children less than 12 years old, geriatric patients older than 65 years old, and in pregnant or nursing women.

Benzaclin is a topical gel consisting of 1% clindamycin (antibiotic) and 5% benzoyl peroxide 5%.

Benzoyl peroxide is added to reduce the likelihood of antibiotic resistance.

<u>Additional useful information</u>

Common side effects of Benzaclin include: skin peeling, redness, dryness, burning, itching and sensitivity to sunlight. These side-effects usually appear at the beginning of treatment and resolve with time. The most common side effect, dry skin, may be treated with a non-allergenic moisturizer.

In general, a patient should see an improvement within the first 2 months of Benzaclin treatment. The usual duration of treatment is 3-4 months.

Interactive Case #49
Pharmacist – Standardized Physician Interaction

Your (Candidate) instructions:

Case description:

You are a pharmacist in a hospital pharmacy. Dr. Robert, a newly hired physician, is waiting in the pharmacy to talk to you. Dr. Robert would like to have detailed information on a new treatment for hepatitis C called Zepatier before prescribing it to his patient. You are expected to educate the physician and help him make a safe prescribing decision. Refer to the physician's introduction and questions, **below**, to fully understand his expectations.

This station must be completed in 7 minutes

Station materials and references:
Compendium of Pharmaceuticals and Specialties (CPS)
Compendium of Therapeutic Choices (CTC)

Standardized physician introductions and questions

"Hi, I am Dr. Robert. I would like to learn about a new product approved for the treatment of hepatitis C called Zepatier. Please, tell me all you know about this product. I am considering prescribing it as monotherapy to my patient who has been diagnosed with hepatitis C."

If the candidate does not explain the benefits of Zepatier, then the standardized physician will ask:

"What are the benefits of Zepatier therapy?"

If the candidate does not list the active ingredients in Zepatier, then the standardized physician will ask:

"What are the active ingredients in Zepatier?"

"Could you explain the mechanism of action?"

If the candidate does not explain the prescribing process, then the standardized physician will ask:

"How is Zepatier prescribed as monotherapy?

If the candidate does not discuss the adverse reactions, then the standardized physician will ask:

"What are potential adverse reactions?"

CASE REVIEW FORM

Write notes, answers, interview and counselling to show how you would solve this case

Solution – Interactive Case #49

Primary goals:

- Educate the physician
- Discuss the active ingredients in Zepatier
- Discuss the benefits of Zepatier therapy
- Discuss the mechanism of action of each active ingredient
- Discuss the prescribing process of Zepatier as monotherapy
- Discuss potential adverse reactions

You are expected to provide the following information to Dr. Robert:

Zepatier is an oral fixed-dose combination tablet consisting of 50 mg elbasvir and 100 mg grazoprevir. Both active ingredients (drugs) are direct-acting antivirals (DAAs). Zepatier is prescribed to adults, alone or with other medications.

Benefits:

The use of DAAs requires shorter treatment duration, much higher cure rates, and fewer side effects

Mechanism of action:
Elbasvir and grazoprevir act synergistically to prevent hepatitis C virus (HCV) from multiplying resulting in a fast reduction of the levels of HCV in the body.
Grazoprevir is an inhibitor of viral serine proteases, encoded by HCV genotypes 1 and 4. These enzymes are essential for viral replication and processing of viral polyproteins into mature proteins.
Elbasvir is an inhibitor of a viral protease essential for viral replication and virion assembly.

Prescribing process:
There are several strains, or genotypes, of HCV (such as genotypes 1 through 6) and there are also subtypes (such as genotype 1a, 1b and so on). Zepatier can be used for between 8 and 16 weeks depending on the patient's HCV genotype and medical history. Zepatier can be used in the following ways:

Zepatier monotherapy
- Patients with genotype 1 or 4 who have not been previously treated – Zepatier treatment lasts for 12 weeks
- Patients with genotype 1 or 4 who have been previously treated with peginterferon and ribavirin and who experienced relapse – Zepatier treatment lasts for 12 weeks

- Patients with genotype 1 who have been previously treated with peginterferon and ribavirin, with or without an HCV protease inhibitor, and who have relapsed – Zepatier treatment lasts for 12 weeks
- Patients with genotype 1b who do not have severe liver injury and who have not been previously treated – Zepatier treatment lasts for 8 weeks
- Patients with genotype 1b who have been previously treated with peginterferon and ribavirin, with or without an HCV protease inhibitor, and who developed virological failure while on therapy – Zepatier treatment lasts for 12 weeks.

Zepatier combination therapies (not required during your interaction with Dr. Robert since he is interested in monotherapy)
With ribavirin:
- Patients with genotype 1a who have previously taken peginterferon and ribavirin, with or without an HCV protease inhibitor, and who developed virological failure while on treatment – Zepatier and ribavirin treatment lasts for 16 weeks
- Patients with genotype 4 who have previously taken peginterferon and ribavirin and who developed virological failure while on treatment – Zepatier and ribavirin treatment lasts for 16 weeks

With sofosbuvir:
- Patients with genotype 3 who have not been previously treated – Zepatier and sofosbuvir (Sovaldi) treatment lasts for 12 weeks

Dosage:
The recommended adult dose of Zepatier is one tablet taken by mouth, once daily. It may be taken with or without food. Swallow the tablet whole with water. Do not crush, chew or break the tablet.

Missed dose:
If a dose is missed, take it as soon as possible and continue with the regular schedule. If it is more than 16 hours since the missed dose, skip the missed dose and continue with the regular dosing schedule. Do not take a double dose to make up for a missed one.

Common adverse reactions:
Unexpected tiredness or lack of energy
Headache
Nausea

Caution:
Avoid in pregnancy. There are no data on the use of Zepatier in pregnant women
Zepatier has not been fully assessed in patients co-infected with hepatitis B and C viruses.

Interactive Case #50
Pharmacist – Standardized Physician Interaction

Your (Candidate) instructions:

Case description:

You are pharmacist in a hospital pharmacy. Dr. Kelvin is waiting in the pharmacy to talk to you. She would like to discuss a new prescription for her patient Ruby Smith for the treatment of type 2 diabetes. Dr. Kelvin is switching Mrs. Smith from glyburide to repaglinide due to a recent episode of hypoglycemia. Repaglinide has lower risk of hypoglycemia compared to glyburide. You are expected to review the prescription and identify any drug related problem(s). Refer to the physician's introduction and questions, **below**, to fully understand her concerns and expectations. You are also expected to record your recommendations and any change(s) on the prescription review sheet.

Patient profile

Name: Ruby Smith
Gender: Female
Age: 57 years old
Medical History: Hyperlipidemia; Type 2 Diabetes
Allergies: Seasonal
Current Medications (Rx & nRx): Glyburide 5 mg po once daily; Gemfibrozil 600 mg po bid; 1 daily multivitamin, Tylenol prn for back pain
Social/lifestyle: Non-smoker, no alcohol intake, physically active – yoga 4 times a week

Station materials and references:
Compendium of Pharmaceuticals and Specialties (CPS)
Compendium of Therapeutic Choices (CTC)
Prescription

This station must be completed in 7 minutes

Prescription

Top Health Hospital
58 Rainy Road
Fall City
777-7777

For: Ruby Smith
Address: 84 High Hill Blvd

                                                    Correct date

Repaglinide 1 mg po once daily

L. Kelvin
_____ Assume signature is correct
L. Kelvin M.D.

Prescription Review Sheet

○ No change, fill the prescription as written

○ Recommended changes as discussed with Dr. Kelvin:

Correct date
Correct pharmacist's identification

Recommended dosage if required:

Standardized physician introductions and questions

"Hi, I am Dr. Kelvin. I have just written this new prescription for my patient Ruby Smith. What would you recommend regarding the prescription?"

If the candidate suggests changing repaglinide without explaining, the standardized physician will ask:

"Could you explain why?"

If the candidate successfully explains that repaglinide interacts with gemfibrozil, then the standardized physician will ask the following 2 questions:

"What is the nature of the interaction?"

"How about changing gemfibrozil instead?"

If the candidate suggests changing gemfibrozil without explaining, the standardized physician will ask the following question:

"Could you explain why?"

If the candidate successfully explains that repaglinide interacts with gemfibrozil, then the standardized physician will ask the following 2 questions:

"What is the nature of the interaction?"

"Could you recommend an alternate cholesterol reducing agent for Ruby?"

It the candidate fails to recommend any changes, the standardized physician will ask:

"Is there any likely drug-drug interaction?"

CASE REVIEW FORM

Write notes, answers, interview and counselling to show how you would solve this case

Solution – Interactive Case #50

Primary goals:

- Identify repaglinide-gemfibrozil interaction
- Explain the nature of the interaction
- Recommend changing gemfibrozil

The candidate is expected to:

Identify repaglinide-gemfibrozil interaction. Gemfibrozil leads to 8-fold increase in repaglinide plasma concentration increasing significantly the risk of severe hypoglycemia. Gemfibrozil and its metabolites inhibit the metabolism of repaglinide.

Recommend changing gemfibrozil. Gemfibrozil belongs to the class of drugs known as fibrates and is used primarily for the reduction of blood triglycerides. It does not have significant effect on the level of total cholesterol.

Recommend a statin as cholesterol reducing agent. Statins are more potent than fibrates.

Interactive case #51: Proper use of Turbuhaler
Pharmacist – Standardized Patient Interaction

Your (Candidate) instructions

Case description:

Mr. Said is 22-year-old male suffering from asthma. His physician is switching him from Flovent to Symbicort to control better his symptoms. He is coming to see the pharmacist (you) with a new prescription for Symbicort 200. He is looking forward to learning from the pharmacist how to properly use his new puffer. Refer to the patient's introduction and questions to fully understand his expectations and concerns.

This station must be completed in 7 minutes

Station materials and references:
Patient profile
Compendium of Pharmaceuticals and Specialties (CPS)
Compendium of Products for Minor Ailments
Symbicort 200 Turbuhaler

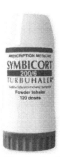

Symbicort Turbuhaler ©Astra Zeneca Inc.

Patient profile

Patient Name: Ahmed Said
Gender: Male
Age: 22 years old
Allergies: None
Medical History: Asthma
Current medications (Rx & nRx): Flovent Diskus 100 ug bid
New prescription: Symbicort 200 2 puffs bid
Social/lifestyle: College student, no alcohol intake, enjoys swimming – at least 3 times weekly

Standardized patient introductions and questions

Case description:

Mr. Said is a 22-year-old male suffering from asthma. His physician is switching him from Flovent to Symbicort to control better his symptoms. He is coming to see the pharmacist (you) with a new prescription for Symbicort 200. He is looking forward to learning from the pharmacist how to properly use his new puffer.

Patient profile

Patient Name: Ahmed Said
Gender: Male
Age: 22 years old
Allergies: None
Medical History: Asthma
Current medications (Rx & nRx): Flovent Diskus 100 ug bid
New prescription: Symbicort 200 2 puffs bid
Social/lifestyle: College student, no alcohol intake, enjoys swimming – at least 3 times weekly

"Hi, I just got this new prescription from my doctor. It is my first time taking this medication and I am not sure how to use it properly. I am also wondering if I can use it if I have a sudden attack"

If not addressed by the candidate after 5 minutes, the standardized patient will ask the following questions:

"Can I use it if I have a sudden attack?"

"What should I do if I forget my medication?"

CASE REVIEW FORM

Write notes, answers, interview and counselling to show how you would solve this case

Solution – Interactive Case #51

<u>Primary goals</u>:

- Educate the patient on how to use Symbicort Turbuhaler
- Confirm that Symbicort can be used for sudden attacks
- Explain how to use Symbicort for sudden attacks

The candidate is expected to:

Discuss the drug schedule with the patient: 2 puffs in the morning and another 2 puffs in the evening.

<u>Note</u>: Symbicort 200 Turbuhaler contains dry powder consisting of 200 µg of budesonide and 6 µg of formoterol per dose. It also contains lactose, which acts as a carrier. The amount added does not normally cause problems in lactose-intolerant patients.

Explain how to use Symbicort Turbuhaler (inhaler):

When you use the inhaler for the first time, or if you have not used it for 7 days or longer, or if the inhaler has been dropped, it may not deliver the right amount of medicine with the first puff. Therefore, before using the inhaler, prime it by spraying the medicine 2 times into the air away from the face, and shake it well for 5 seconds before each spray.

Directions:

- Take the inhaler out of the moisture-protective foil pouch before you use it for the first time.
- Prime the inhaler before use by shaking the inhaler well for 5 seconds and then releasing a test spray. Once again, shake the inhaler and release a second test spray.
- Breathe out to the end of a normal breath (exhale). Do not breathe into the inhaler.
- Holding the inhaler leveled, put the mouthpiece fully into your mouth and close your lips around it. Do not block the mouthpiece with your teeth or tongue.
- While pressing down firmly and fully on the grey top of the inhaler, breathe in through your mouth as deeply as you can until you have taken a full deep breath.
- Hold your breath and remove the mouthpiece from your mouth. Continue holding your breath as long as you can up to 10 seconds before breathing out slowly. This gives the medicine time to settle in your airways and lungs.
- Release your finger from the top and then turn your head away from the inhaler. Breathe out slowly to the end of a normal breath. Do not breathe into the inhaler.
- Shake the inhaler again for 5 seconds and take the second puff following exactly the same steps you used for the first puff.
- Replace the mouthpiece cover after using the medicine.

Gargle and rinse your mouth with water after each dose to help prevent hoarseness, throat irritation, and infection in the mouth. Do not swallow the water after rinsing.

Discard the inhaler after you have used the number of inhalations on the product label and box, or within 3 months of opening the foil pouch. Your inhaler is empty and should be thrown out when the zero or a red line is in the centre of the dose-counting window.

Clean the inhaler twice weekly by wiping the mouthpiece with dry cloth. Never wash the mouthpiece. However, you must use a new inhaler with each refill of your medicine.

If you miss a dose, take it as soon as possible. However, if it is almost time for the next dose, skip the missed dose and go back to regular dosing schedule. Do not double the dose.

Confirm that Symbicort can be used to relief sudden asthma attacks. Symbicort works by decreasing the frequency and severity of asthma attacks, and it can be used as a reliever medication for sudden asthma attacks. For fast relief, use 1 additional inhalation as needed and repeat after a few minutes (to a maximum of 6 inhalations) if symptoms persist. The maximum recommended total daily dose is 8 inhalations.

Discuss common side effects:
- Body aches or pain
- Chills
- Cough, fever, sneezing, or sore throat
- Ear congestion
- Fever
- Headache
- Loss of voice
- Stuffy or runny nose
- Chest tightness

This medication may cause fungus infection of the mouth or throat (thrush). Tell your doctor right away if you have white patches in the mouth or throat, or pain when eating or swallowing. Do not stop using this medication without telling your doctor.

Store at room temperature, away from heat and direct light. Do not freeze. Do not keep this medicine inside a car where it could be exposed to extreme heat or cold. Store the turbuhaler with the mouthpiece down.

Discuss non-pharmacologic strategies:
- Avoid known triggers such as air pollution, dust, cigarette smoke, mold, pollens
- Avoid extreme weather: cold air, dry air
- Avoid stress
- Encourage the patient to continue swimming. Swimming is a healthy form of aerobic exercise for people with asthma.

Summarize and assess patient understanding

Interactive case #52: Proper use of Repatha SureClick Autoinjector
Pharmacist – Standardized Patient Interaction

Your (Candidate) instructions

Case description:

Mr. Gill is a 52-year-old male suffering from heterozygous familial hypercholesterolemia (HeFH). His LDL-cholesterol levels are still above normal range despite several months of dietary modifications and Lipitor therapy at maximum tolerated dose. His hepatic and renal functions are normal. His physician prescribes Repatha as an additional LDL-cholesterol lowering strategy. Mr. Gill is visiting your pharmacy to fill his new prescription. He is expecting to learn from you how to properly use Repatha SureClick Autoinjector. Refer to the patient's introduction and questions to fully understand his expectations and concerns.

This station must be completed in 7 minutes

Station materials and references: Patient profile
Compendium of Pharmaceuticals and Specialties (CPS)
Repatha SureClick Autoinjector

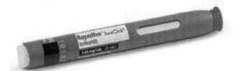

Repatha Single-Use SureClick AutoInjector ©Amgen Inc.

Patient profile

Patient Name: Sunny Gill
Gender: Male
Age: 52 years old
Allergies: None
Medical History: Arthritis in the left knee, Heterozygous Familial Hypercholesterolemia
Current medications (Rx & nRx): Lipitor 80 mg once daily, Tylenol 500 mg bid, daily multivitamin, Omega-3 supplement
New prescription: Repatha 140 mg SC q2weeks
Social/lifestyle: University Professor, no alcohol intake, plays table tennis, enjoys walking – at least 5 times weekly

Standardized patient introductions and questions

Case description:

Mr. Gill is a 52-year-old male suffering from heterozygous familial hypercholesterolemia (HeFH). His LDL-cholesterol level is still above normal range despite several months of dietary modifications and Lipitor therapy at maximum tolerated dose. His hepatic and renal functions are normal. His physician prescribes Repatha as an additional LDL-cholesterol lowering strategy. Mr. Gill is visiting your pharmacy to fill his new prescription. He is expecting to learn from you how to properly use Repatha SureClick Autoinjector.

Patient profile

Patient Name: Sunny Gill
Gender: Male
Age: 52 years old
Allergies: None
Medical History: Arthritis in the left knee, Heterozygous Familial Hypercholesterolemia
Current medications (Rx & nRx): Lipitor 60 mg once daily, Tylenol 500 mg bid, daily multivitamin, Omega-3 supplement
New prescription: Repatha 140 mg SC q2weeks
Social/lifestyle: University Professor, no alcohol intake, plays table tennis, enjoys walking – at least 5 times weekly

"Hi, I just got this new prescription from my doctor. It is my first time taking this medication and I am not sure how to use and store it properly. I would like also to learn about the side effects of the medication"

If not addressed by the candidate after 5 minutes, the standardized patient will ask the following questions:

"What are the side effects?"

"What is the best way to store it?"

"What should I do if I forget my medication?"

CASE REVIEW FORM

Write notes, answers, interview and counselling to show how you would solve this case

Solution – Interactive Case #52

<u>Primary goals</u>:

- Educate the patient on how to use Repatha SureClick Autoinjector
- Discuss side effects
- Discuss proper storage

The candidate is expected to:

Discuss the drug schedule with the patient: 1 subcutaneous injection every two weeks.

Explain how to use Repatha SureClick Autoinjector:

Remove 1 Repatha SureClick autoinjector from the refrigerator at least 30 minutes before injecting; it helps administer the entire dose and minimize injection discomfort.

Repatha may take longer to inject if it has not reached room temperature. Do not heat the autoinjector. Do not try to warm the autoinjector by using a heat source such as hot water or microwave. Let it warm up on its own.

Do not shake the Repatha SureClick autoinjector

Do not remove the orange cap from the Repatha SureClick autoinjector until you are ready to inject.

Do not leave the autoinjector in direct sunlight

Inspect the Repatha SureClick autoinjector. Make sure the medicine in the window is clear and colorless to slightly yellow.
- Do not use if the medicine is cloudy or discolored or contains particles
- Do not use if any part appears cracked or broken
- Do not use if the autoinjector has been dropped
- Do not use if the orange cap is missing or not securely attached.
- Do not use if the product is expired

Wash your hands thoroughly with soap and water

Clean the injection site with alcohol wipe and let dry. Do not touch the area before injecting.

Do not inject in areas of skin that are bruised, red, tender, or hard. Avoid injecting in scars or stretch marks. Rotate administration sites

Recommended administration sites

Self-injection: Thigh or abdomen (except for the 2-inch area around the naval)
Caregiver: Thigh, abdomen, or outer area of upper arm

Pull the orange cap off only when you are ready to inject. Do not leave the orange cap off for more than five minutes. This can dry out the medicine.
- Do not twist, bend, or wiggle the orange cap
- Do not put the orange cap back onto the autoinjector

Stretch or pinch the injection site to create a firm surface.
Thigh
Stretch method: Stretch the skin firmly by moving your thumb and fingers in opposite directions, creating an area about two inches wide.
Stomach or upper arm
Pinch method: Pinch the skin firmly between your thumb and fingers, creating an area about two inches wide.

Keep skin stretched or pinched while injecting

Hold the stretched or pinched skin. With the orange cap off, place the yellow end of the autoinjector on the skin at 90 degrees. Do not touch the gray start button yet. Firmly push down the autoinjector onto the skin until it stops moving. You must push all the way down but do not touch the gray start button until you are ready to inject.

When you are ready to inject, press the gray start button. You will hear a click. Keep pushing the autoinjector down on your skin. Then lift your thumb while still holding the autoinjector on your skin. Your injection could take about 15 seconds.

Window turns from clear to yellow when the injection is done. You may hear a second click.

After you remove the autoinjector from your skin, the needle will be automatically covered.
Important: When you remove the autoinjector, if the window has not turned yellow, or if it looks like the medicine is still injecting, this means you have not received a full dose. Call your healthcare provider immediately.

Throw away the used autoinjector and orange needle cap. Put the used autoinjector and orange needle cap in a sharps disposal container right away after use. Do not dispose of the autoinjector or orange cap in your household trash. When your sharps disposal container is almost full, you will need to follow your community guidelines for the right way to dispose. Do not dispose of your used sharps disposal container in your household trash. Do not recap the autoinjector or put fingers into the yellow safety guard.
Important: Always keep the sharps disposal container out of reach of children.

Check the injection site. If there is blood, press a cotton ball or gauze pad on your injection site. Apply an adhesive bandage if needed. Do not rub the injection site.

Most common adverse effect is nasopharyngitis

Missed Dose

Administer as soon as possible if there are more than 7 days until the next scheduled dose, otherwise omit the missed dose and administer the next dose according to the original schedule.

Storage

- Refrigerate at 2-8°C (36-46°F) in original package
- Alternatively, you may store at room temperature (20-25°C) in original package; however, under these conditions, drug must be used within 30 days; if not used within the 30 days, discard.
- Do not freeze the Repatha SureClick autoinjector or use a Repatha SureClick
- autoinjector that has been frozen.
- Protect from direct light
- Do not expose to temperatures >25°C
- Do not shake

Discuss non-pharmacologic strategies:

- Advise the patient to follow-up with his physician within 4-8 weeks for blood cholesterol monitoring to evaluate his response to Repatha
- Encourage the patient to continue exercising
- Encourage the patient to remain compliant with healthy diet

Summarize and assess patient understanding

Additional learning: Mechanism of action of Repatha

Evolocumab (trade name Repatha) is a monoclonal antibody. Evolocumab is a full human monoclonal antibody that inhibits proprotein convertase subtilisin/kexin type 9 (PCSK9). PCSK9 is a protein that targets LDL receptors for degradation and thereby reduces the liver's ability to remove LDL-cholesterol from the blood.

Interactive case #53: Recreational Cannabis
Pharmacist – Standardized Patient Interaction

Your (Candidate) instructions

Case description:

Jason Clark is considering using recreational cannabis. Jason is visiting the pharmacy to have as much information as possible on recreational cannabis. His primary concern is safety. He seems to be overwhelmed by the information on the internet. He is confident that the pharmacist will help. Refer to the patient's introduction and questions to fully understand his expectations and concerns.

This station must be completed in 7 minutes

Station materials and references:

Patient profile
Compendium of Pharmaceuticals and Specialties (CPS 2019)

Patient profile

Patient Name: Jason Clark
Gender: Male
Age: 29 years old
Allergies: None
Medical History: None
Current medications (Rx & nRx): None
Other: One daily multivitamin
Social/lifestyle: College instructor, non-smoker, occasional alcohol intake with friends, physically active – visits the gym 5 times a week

Standardized patient introduction and questions

Case description:
Jason Clark is considering using recreational cannabis. Jason is visiting the pharmacy to have as much information as possible on recreational cannabis. His primary concern is safety. He seems to be overwhelmed by the information on the internet. He is confident that the pharmacist will help. Refer to the patient's introduction and questions to fully understand his expectations and concerns.

Patient profile

Patient Name: Jason Clark
Gender: Male
Age: 29 years old
Allergies: None
Medical History: None
Current medications (Rx & nRx): None
Other: One daily multivitamin
Social/lifestyle: College instructor, non-smoker, occasional alcohol intake with friends, physically active – visits the gym 5 times a week

"Hi, I am thinking about using recreational cannabis. I would like to learn as much as possible about cannabis. My main concern is safety. How to use it? What to expect?"

CASE REVIEW FORM

Write notes, answers, interview and counselling to show how you would solve this case

Solution – Interactive Case #53

<u>Primary goals</u>:
- Determine if cannabis is appropriate for the client.
- Provide patient education if cannabis is appropriate.
- Emphasis that smoking is not recommended and explain why.

The candidate is expected to:
First, refer to the profile and ask questions to determine whether the client should avoid cannabis or not by following the guidelines below.
Generally, avoid using cannabis in patients:
- younger than 25
- with a strong family history of psychosis or schizophrenia
- with current or past cannabis use disorder or other substance use disorder (e.g., alcohol, benzodiazepine, opioids)
- who are pregnant, planning to become pregnant or breastfeeding
- with known allergy to cannabis, THC, CBD or any other cannabinoid

Use cannabis with caution in patients with current or past history of anxiety or mood disorder.
<u>Note</u>: CUDIT-R tool or CAGE tool can be used in practice to screen for risk of substance abuse.
Second, provide comprehensive patient education if cannabis is appropriate.

Common methods of use
Inhaled cannabis starts working within 10 min and effects last 2-4h (up to 24h)
Oral cannabis (e.g. oils, edibles) starts working at around 1h and effects last 4-6h (up to 24h)
Vaping and edibles likely safer than smoking. Smoking is associated with increased risk of respiratory damage.
<u>Note:</u> Cannabis can be smoked, vaporized, taken orally, sublingually, topically or rectally. Different routes of administration will result in different pharmacokinetic and pharmacodynamic properties of the drug.
Currently, cannabis edibles are not legally available for purchase.

How to reduce cannabis related harm?
Avoid driving for several hours after use
Avoid smoking cannabis to reduce risk of respiratory adverse effect
Keep away from children, especially edibles
Delay age of first use as long as possible

The most common adverse effects are:
- Being very happy
- Sedation
- Relaxation
- Difficulty speaking
- Numbness
- Disconnected thoughts
- Muscle twitching
- Changes in heart rate and blood pressure

Dosing
Effects vary considerably based on strain
Start with lower THC, less than 9%
Average use is 1.5- 3g of herbal cannabis/day
1 joint ≈ 0.5g of cannabis
Inhaled: start with 1 puff and wait 10 min to assess effect, repeat as needed
Edible: start with 1 small bite and wait 1 hour to assess effect, repeat as needed

How to manage cannabis adverse effects?
- Start cannabinoids at a low dose, and gradually increase
- Reduce dose (frequency, potency, amount) or stop
- Select a strain with lower THC to reduce cognitive side effects
- Stop if signs of cannabis use disorder are experienced. These signs include lack of motivation, poor work/study performance, problematic relationships
- Withdrawal symptoms include anxiety, irritability, anger, sleep disturbance, fatigue, cannabis craving, restlessness

Since Jason takes alcohol occasionally, it is important to mention that Cannabis has additive CNS effects (sedation, dizziness…) with alcohol. Avoid alcohol and cannabis combination.
Summarize and assess patient understanding

Interactive case #54: Prescription Cannabinoid for Neuropathic Pain
Pharmacist – Standardized Patient Interaction

Your (Candidate) instructions

Case description:

Ms. Bob is a 67 years female patient suffering from Multiple Sclerosis (MS). She has been also diagnosed with MS associated neuropathic pain. Ms. Bob presents to the pharmacy with a new prescription for Nabiximols. She has some questions and concerns regarding the use of the medication. Please, provide your assistance.

This station must be completed in 7 minutes

Station materials and references:

Patient profile
Compendium of Pharmaceuticals and Specialties (CPS)

Patient profile

Patient Name: Marilyn Bob
Gender: Female
Age: 67 years old
Allergies: Seasonal
Medical History: Social anxiety, high blood cholesterol, multiple sclerosis diagnosed 3 years ago
Current medications (Rx & nRx): Fluoxetine capsule 20 mg po daily, Rosuvastatin 20 mg po daily, Teriflunomide 14 mg tab po daily, Tylenol prn for headaches
New prescription: Nabiximols 1 spray sl hs then increase by 1 spray daily until 6 sprays daily, 1 spray sl q4h
Social/lifestyle: Retired teacher, non-smoker, no alcohol intake

Note: The standardized patient shows some signs of shyness including avoidance of eye contact.

Standardized patient introduction and questions

Case description:
Ms. Bob is a 67 years female patient suffering from Multiple Sclerosis (MS). She has been also diagnosed with MS associated neuropathic pain. Ms. Bob presents to the pharmacy with a new prescription for Nabiximols. She has some questions and concerns regarding the use of the medication. Please, provide your assistance.

Patient profile

Patient Name: Marilyn Bob
Gender: Female
Age: 67 years old
Allergies: Seasonal
Medical History: Social anxiety, high blood cholesterol, multiple sclerosis diagnosed 3 years ago
Current medications (Rx & nRx): Fluoxetine capsule 20 mg po daily, Rosuvastatin 20 mg po daily, Teriflunomide 14 mg tab po daily, Tylenol prn for headaches
New prescription: Nabiximols 1 spray sl hs then increase by 1 spray daily until 6 sprays daily, 1 spray sl q4h
Social/lifestyle: Retired teacher, non-smoker, no alcohol intake

"Hi, I just got this new prescription from my physician. It is my first time taking this medication and I am not sure how to use it. Could you also tell me what to expect? How different is it from cannabis?"

Note: the standardized patient shows some signs of shyness including avoidance of eye contact.

If not addressed by the candidate after 4 minutes, the standardized patient will ask the following questions:
How do I take this medication?

What should I expect while taking this medication? Should I be concerned about grogginess?
How different is this medication from cannabis?

CASE REVIEW FORM

Write notes, answers, interview and counselling to show how you would solve this case

Solution – Interactive Case #54

Primary goals:
- Discuss the administration instructions of Nabiximols
- Discuss the differences between Nabiximols and Cannabis
- Discuss the adverse effects of Nabiximols including drowsiness
- Initiate follow up to monitor the patient's anxiety and drowsiness. Anxiety has been associated with the use of cannabinoids. Fluoxetine can induce drowsiness resulting in additive effect with Nabiximols.

The candidate is expected to:

Refer to the profile and ask questions to determine whether the client should avoid cannabis or not by following the guidelines below.
Generally, avoid using cannabis in patients:
- younger than 25
- with a strong family history of psychosis or schizophrenia
- with current or past cannabis use disorder or other substance use disorder (e.g., alcohol, benzodiazepine, opioids)
- who are pregnant, planning to become pregnant or breastfeeding
- with known allergy to cannabis, THC, CBD or any other cannabinoid

Use cannabis with caution in patients with current or past history of anxiety or mood disorder. The patient suffers from anxiety.
Nabiximols (Sativex) is a prescription cannabinoid that contains extracted THC and CBD; 2.7 mg THC and 2.5 mg CBD per spray. Nabiximols is preferred over cannabis due to efficient dosing. Cannabis contains over 400 different compounds.

Administration Instructions
Refrigerate prior to dispensing
Device requires priming:
1. Shake the vial gently before use
2. Remove the protective cap
3. Hold the vial in an upright position, then prime by pressing on the actuator two or three times firmly and quickly, directing into a tissue until a fine spray appears

Normal use:
1. Shake the vial gently
2. Remove the protective cap
3. Hold the vial in upright position and direct into the mouth
4. Press firmly and quickly towards the buccal surface in the following areas: below the tongue or inside the cheeks. You should alternate sides. Never aim at the throat, Nabiximols can cause irritation
5. Replace the protective cap
6. Keep away from heat and direct sunlight

Dosage

On day 1, 1 spray sublingually at bedtime then increase the dose by 1 spray daily to a maximum of 6 sprays daily. Sprays must be spread evenly during the day.

Storage

Store the vial upright in the refrigerator (2-8°C) prior to opening. Do not freeze.
Once the vial is opened it may be stored at room temperature (15-25°C)
Once opened and in use, Nabiximols should be used within 42 days.

Side effects

Common side effects are mild to moderate and mainly consist of either application site reactions in the mouth such as dry mouth or stinging, or intoxication reactions such as dizziness, drowsiness, disorientation or impaired memory.
Discuss non-pharmacologic options such as massage, physical activity and acupuncture
Summarize and confirm that patient understands

Interactive case #55: Chemotherapy induced nausea and vomiting
Pharmacist – Standardized Physician Interaction

Your (Candidate) instructions:

Case description:

Dr. Ali is waiting in the pharmacy to talk to you, the pharmacist on duty in a hospital pharmacy. He is seeking your guidance to prescribe a trial of cannabinoid to his patient Jim for the treatment of nausea and vomiting induced by chemotherapy. Jim is already on two antiemetics. You are expected to recommend a prescription cannabinoid and provide relevant prescribing information. Refer to the physician's introduction and questions, below, to fully understand his expectations and concerns.

Station references: Compendium of Pharmaceuticals and Specialties (CPS)

This station must be completed in <u>7 minutes</u>

Patient profile

Name: Jim Young
Gender: Male
Age: 55 years old
Medical History: lung cancer, hyperlipidemia
Allergies: None
Current Medications (Rx & nRx): Atorvastatin 40 mg daily, Chemotherapy for lung cancer
Social/lifestyle: Business owner, stopped smoking 4 years ago, no alcohol intake, he has been on low fat diet since his hyperlipidemia diagnosis, physically active – 5 times weekly

Standardized physician introduction and questions

"Hi, I am Dr. Ali. I would like your guidance to prescribe a trial of cannabinoid to my Jim Young to manage his nausea and vomiting induced by chemotherapy. Jim is already on two antiemetics. without Which prescription cannabinoid would you recommend? What would be the recommended dose? Jim is cannabinoid naïve."

If the candidate suggests a cannabinoid other than Nabilone, the standardized physician will ask:
"Is this the most recommended cannabinoid for chemotherapy induced nausea and vomiting?"

If the candidate answers "yes", then the standardized physician will ask:
"How about Nabilone?"

If the candidate recommends Nabilone, the standardized physician must ask:
"What are the most common adverse effects?"

"What are the active compounds in Nabilone"

"What are other indications of Nabilone?"

CASE REVIEW FORM

Write notes, answers, interview and counselling to show how you would solve this case

Solution – Interactive Case #55

<u>Primary goal</u>:

Recommend adjunctive treatment of Nabilone 1 mg twice a day the night before his chemotherapy cycle.
The candidate is expected to provide the following information:
- Nabilone (Cesamet) is synthetic THC analogue
- Usually dose is 1-2mg po BID for CINV. 1 mg would be more appropriate for Jim who is cannabis naive.
- Cannabinoids are the most effective persistent chemotherapy induced nausea and vomiting (CINV) when used as adjunctive treatment. Of all the cannabinoids, including cannabis, nabilone has the strongest evidence
- Common side effects are mild to moderate intoxication reactions such as dizziness, drowsiness, disorientation or impaired memory

Other indications of Nabilone
off-label: AIDS-related anorexia, palliative pain and neuropathic pain

Non Interactive Case #1: Prescription Labels Check

Candidate instructions:

Identify any mistakes, omissions or concerns on each prescription label. Assume each prescription is correct and omission of auxiliary labels, pharmacy contact information or practitioner ID is not to be considered a mistake.
Use your answer sheet to record your answers. You have a total of **4 prescriptions** in this station.
Station Reference: CPS - Compendium of Pharmaceuticals and Specialties

You have 7 minutes to complete this station

Written Rx 1

```
Rx 1
Patient Name: Haley James
Address: 3545 Hillcrest Street

                                                Correct date

        Lomotil 2.5 mg
        PO ii tabs tid for diarrhea
        Mitte: 7 days

    T June
    _____        Assume signature is correct
        T. June M.D.
```

Dispensed Rx 1 label

```
Rx 1                                    Dr. T. June
Haley James
                                        Correct date

        Take three tablets orally three times a
        day for diarrhea for seven days

        Lomotil 25 mg
        42 tablets
```

Written Rx 2

Rx 2
Patient Name: Rosie Pearson
Address: 7-500 Sunny Bay

                                                      Correct date

Sutent 50 mg
PO 50 mg cap qd x 4 wk followed by 2 wk off treatment, then repeat for 6 wk

K. Said
_____ Assume signature is correct
K. Said M.D.

Dispensed Rx 2 label

Rx 2   Dr. K. Said
Rosie Pearson
                                              Correct date

Take one tablet orally once a day for four weeks
Follow with two weeks off treatment
Then take one tablet orally once a day for six weeks

Sutent 50 mg
84 tablets

Written Rx 3

```
Rx 3
Patient Name: Ryan Timmy
Address: 3590 3rd Road

                                          Correct date

         Detrol 1 mg tab
         PO 2 mg bid for overactive bladder
         Mitte: 120 tabs



       P. Sean
   _____   Assume signature is correct
        P. Sean M.D.
```

Dispensed Rx 3 label

```
Rx 3                              Dr. P. Sean
Ryan Timmy
                                  Correct date


         Take two tablets orally twice a day for
         overactive bladder for 30 days

         Detrol 1 mg
         120 tablets
```

Written Rx 4

Rx 4
Patient Name: Thomas Summer
Address: 9999 Hill Street

                                                               Correct date

Aricept 10 mg
PO i tab qd for dementia
Mitte: 90 days

B. Bernard
_____ Assume signature is correct
B. Bernard M.D.

Dispensed Rx 4 label

Rx 4   Dr. D. Bernard
Thomas Simmar
                                                   Correct date

Take two tablets orally once a day for
dementia for 90 days

Aricept 5 mg
180 tablets

Answer Sheet: Prescription Labels Check

Rx 1	Is this prescription label consistent with the prescription? Yes　　　　　　　No What would you correct?
Rx 2	Is this prescription label consistent with the prescription? Yes　　　　　　　No What would you correct?
Rx 3	Is this prescription label consistent with the prescription? Yes　　　　　　　No What would you correct?
Rx 4	Is this prescription label consistent with the prescription? Yes　　　　　　　No What would you correct?

Answer Key #1

Rx 1	Is this prescription label consistent with the prescription? No What would you correct? Wrong instructions Wrong drug strength
Rx 2	Is this prescription label consistent with the prescription? No What would you correct? Wrong drug form (cap not tab) Wrong number of capsules (70 capsules)
Rx 3	Is this prescription label consistent with the prescription? Yes What would you correct?
Rx 4	Is this prescription label consistent with the prescription? No What would you correct? Wrong patient name Wrong physician initial

Non Interactive Case #2: Prescription Labels Check

Candidate instructions:

Identify any mistakes, omissions or concerns on each prescription label. Assume each prescription is correct and omission of auxiliary labels, pharmacy contact information or practitioner ID is not to be considered a mistake.
Use your answer sheet to record your answers. You have a total of **4 prescriptions** in this station.
Station Reference: CPS – Compendium of Pharmaceuticals and Specialties

You have 7 minutes to complete this station

Written Rx 1

> Rx 1
> Patient Name: Miranda Douglas
> Address: 511 Victoria Street
>
>   Correct date
>
> Xeloda 500 mg
> PO i tab q12h for 2 weeks for breast cancer followed by 1 week off treatment, then repeat treatment for 2 weeks
>
> *L. Junior*
> _____ Assume signature is correct
>   L. Junior M.D.

Dispensed Rx 1 label

> Rx 1   Dr. L. Junior
> Miranda Douglas
>   Correct date
>
> Take one tablet orally every twelve hours for two weeks for breast cancer followed by one week off treatment
> Then take one tablet orally every twelve hours for two weeks
>
> Xeloda 500 mg
> 56 tablets

Written Rx 2

Rx 2
Patient Name: Bob Singh
Address: 4001 Simon Fraser Road

                                                      Correct date

Ceftin
PO 500 mg bid x 7 days

M Hamed
_____ Assume signature is correct
M. Hamed M.D.

Dispensed Rx 2 label

Rx 2   Dr. M. Hamed
Bob Song
                                Correct date

Take one tablet orally twice a day
for 7 days

Ceftin 500 mg
18 tablets

Written Rx 3

```
Rx 3
Patient Name: Pauline Maison
Address: 444B Crescent

                                                    Correct date


    Keppra
    Start PO 500 mg bid increase by 500 mg bid q2wk until 3000 mg
    daily then continue for 2 weeks



       H. Tremblay
    _____      Assume signature is correct
       H. Tremblay M.D.
```

Dispensed Rx 3 label

```
Rx 3                                       Dr. H. Tramdley
Pauline Maison
                                             Correct date

          Take one tablet orally twice a day for two
          weeks
          Then take two tablets orally twice a day
          for two weeks
          Then take three tablets orally twice a day
          for two weeks

          Keppra 500 mg
          168 tablets
```

Written Rx 4

```
Rx 4
Patient Name: Fanny Rock
Address: 7775 Hill Place

                                          Correct date

           Effexor XR 37.5mg
           i cap daily for anxiety
           Mitte: 100 capsules




            K. Sunny
    _____    Assume signature is correct
          K. Sunny M.D.
```

Dispensed Rx 4 label

```
Rx 4                              Dr. K. Sunny
Fanny Rock
                                  Correct date


        Take one tablet twice a day for
        anxiety for 100 days

        Effexor XR 3.75mg
        100 tablets
```

Answer Sheet: Prescription Labels Check

Rx 1	Is this prescription label consistent with the prescription? Yes　　　　　　　　No What would you correct?
Rx 2	Is this prescription label consistent with the prescription? Yes　　　　　　　　No What would you correct?
Rx 3	Is this prescription label consistent with the prescription? Yes　　　　　　　　No What would you correct?
Rx 4	Is this prescription label consistent with the prescription? Yes　　　　　　　　No What would you correct?

Answer Key #2

Rx 1	Is this prescription label consistent with the prescription? Yes What would you correct?
Rx 2	Is this prescription label consistent with the prescription? No What would you correct? Patient name Wrong number of tablets (14 tablets)
Rx 3	Is this prescription label consistent with the prescription? No What would you correct? Physician name
Rx 4	Is this prescription label consistent with the prescription? No What would you correct? Wrong instructions Wrong drug strength

Non Interactive Case #3: Prescription Labels Check

Candidate instructions:

Identify any mistakes, omissions or concerns on each prescription label. Assume each prescription is correct and omission of auxiliary labels, pharmacy contact information or practitioner ID is not to be considered a mistake.
Use your answer sheet to record your answers. You have a total of **4 prescriptions** in this station.
Station Reference: CPS – Compendium of Pharmaceuticals and Specialties

You have 7 minutes to complete this station

Written Rx 1

```
Rx 1
Patient Name: Paula Anderson
Address: 522A Fall Street

                                              Correct date

         Levaquin 500 mg
         PO 500 mg q24h x 10 days for infection


         K. Kim
         _____    Assume signature is correct
         K. Kim M.D.
```

Dispensed Rx 1 label

```
Rx 1                                    Dr. K. Kim
Paula Anderson
                                        Correct date

         Take two tablets orally every twenty-four
         hours for ten days for Community-
         Acquired Pneumonia

         Levaquin 250 mg
         20 tablets
```

Written Rx 2

> Rx 2
> Patient Name: Ali Karim
> Address: 991 Highview Street
>
>   Correct date
>
> Zithromax 100 mg/5 ml suspension
> PO 10 mg/kg on day one, then 5 mg/kg for 4 more days (max: 250 mg/day) for bacterial infection. Child weight = 28kg
>
> *D. Johnson*
> _____ Assume signature is correct
>   D. Johnson M.D.

Dispensed Rx 2 label

> Rx 2   Dr. D. Johnson
> Ali Karim
>   Correct date
>
>   Take 12.5 ml orally on day one
>   Then take 7 ml daily for four more days
>   for bacterial infection
>
>   Zithromax 100mg/5ml suspension

Written Rx 3

```
Rx 3
Patient Name: Mirna Hamid
Address: 8 Chateau Place

                                        Correct date

        Abilify 15 mg
        PO i tab qd x 5 weeks for schizophrenia


        S. Samuel
    _____    Assume signature is correct
        S. Samuel M.D.
```

Dispensed Rx 3 label

```
Rx 3                              Dr. S. Samuel
Mirna Hamid
                                  Correct date


        Take one tablet orally once a day for
        Five weeks for schizophrenia

    Abilify 15 mg
    35 tablets
```

Written Rx 4

Rx 4
Patient Name: Cynthia Smith
Address: 675 Hill Way

                                        Correct date

Lyrica 75 mg
150 mg daily in 2 divided doses for neuropathic pain
Mitte: 90 days

Y. Lee

_____ Assume signature is correct
Y. Lee M.D.

Dispensed Rx 4 label

Rx 4   Dr. Y Lee
Cynthia Smith
                                      Correct date

Take one tablet twice a day for
90 days for neuropathic pain

Lyrica 75 mg
180 tablets

Answer Sheet: Prescription Labels Check

Rx 1	Is this prescription label consistent with the prescription? Yes No What would you correct?
Rx 2	Is this prescription label consistent with the prescription? Yes No What would you correct?
Rx 3	Is this prescription label consistent with the prescription? Yes No What would you correct?
Rx 4	Is this prescription label consistent with the prescription? Yes No What would you correct?

Answer Key #3

Rx 1	Is this prescription label consistent with the prescription? Yes What would you correct?
Rx 2	Is this prescription label consistent with the prescription? Yes What would you correct?
Rx 3	Is this prescription label consistent with the prescription? Yes What would you correct?
Rx 4	Is this prescription label consistent with the prescription? Yes What would you correct?

Non Interactive Case #4: Prescription Labels Check

Candidate instructions:

Identify any mistakes, omissions or concerns on each prescription label. Assume each prescription is correct and omission of auxiliary labels, pharmacy contact information or practitioner ID is not to be considered a mistake.
Use your answer sheet to record your answers. You have a total of **5 prescriptions** in this station.
Station Reference: CPS – Compendium of Pharmaceuticals and Specialties

You have 7 minutes to complete this station

Written Rx 1

```
Rx 1
Patient Name: Hanna Ryan
Address: 88C Winter Street

                                             Correct date

        Onglyza 5mg
        PO one tablet daily for diabetes
        Mitte:  120 days

      N. Wong
   _____     Assume signature is correct
        N. Wong M.D.
```

Dispensed Rx 1 label

```
Rx 1                               Dr. N. Wamg
Hanna Ryan
                                   Correct date


        Take one tablet orally once a day
             for 120 days for diabetes

        Omglysa 50mg
        120 capsules
```

Written Rx 2

```
Rx 2
Patient Name: Yan Lee
Address: 350 Hall Street

                                          Correct date

            Invirase 200 mg
            5 caps bid for HIV infection
            Mitte: 8 weeks

         K. Mason
      _____   Assume signature is correct
         K. Mason M.D.
```

Dispensed Rx 2 label

```
Rx 2                                    Dr. K. Mason
Yan Lee
                                        Correct date


         Take five tablets twice a day for nine
         weeks for HIV infection

      Invirase 200 mg
      560 tablets
```

Written Rx 3

```
Rx 3
Patient Name: April Park
Address: 35 Oak Bay

                                          Correct date


          Cozaar 50 mg
          One tablet daily for high blood pressure
          Mitte: 120 tablets

     G. Ali
     _____    Assume signature is correct
          G. Ali M.D.
```

Dispensed Rx 3 label

```
Rx 3                            Dr. G. Ali
April Bark
                                Correct date


          Take two tablets once a week for
          for 130 days for high blood pressure

     Cozzar 25 mg
     120 tablets
```

Written Rx 4

> Rx 4
> Patient Name: David Olsen
> Address: 442 2nd Street
>
> Correct date
>
> Valtrex 500 mg
> PO 500 mg bid x 3 days for recurrent genital herpes
>
> *O.Albanny*
> _____ Assume signature is correct
> O. Albanny M.D.

Dispensed Rx 4 label

> Rx 4   Dr. O. Albanny
> David Olsen
>   Correct date
>
> Take one tablet twice a day for
> 5 days for recurrent genital herpes
>
> Valtrex 50 mg
> 10 tablets

Written Rx 5

```
Rx 5
Patient Name: Miranda Josef
Address: 35 Canada Way

                                          Correct date


    Brilinta 90 mg
    One tablet bid x 60 days


      W. George
    _____  Assume signature is correct
       W. George M.D.
```

Dispensed Rx 5 label

```
Rx 5                              Dr. W. George
Miranda Josef
                                  Correct date


       Take one tablet twice a day for 60 days

       Brilinta 90 mg
       120 tablets
```

Answer Sheet: Prescription Labels Check

Rx 1	Is this prescription label consistent with the prescription? Yes No What would you correct?
Rx 2	Is this prescription label consistent with the prescription? Yes No What would you correct?
Rx 3	Is this prescription label consistent with the prescription? Yes No What would you correct?
Rx 4	Is this prescription label consistent with the prescription? Yes No What would you correct?
Rx 5	Is this prescription label consistent with the prescription? Yes No What would you correct?

Answer Key #4

Rx 1	Is this prescription label consistent with the prescription? No What would you correct? Wrong drug name Wrong drug strength Wrong drug form Wrong physician name
Rx 2	Is this prescription label consistent with the prescription? No What would you correct? Wrong duration of treatment Wrong drug form (capsules not tablets)
Rx 3	Is this prescription label consistent with the prescription? No What would you correct? Wrong patient name Wrong duration of treatment Wrong instructions
Rx 4	Is this prescription label consistent with the prescription? No What would you correct? Wrong duration of treatment Wrong drug strength Wrong number of tablets
Rx 5	Is this prescription label consistent with the prescription? Yes What would you correct?

Non Interactive Case #5: Prescription Labels Check

Candidate instructions:

Identify any mistakes, omissions or concerns on each prescription label. Assume each prescription is correct and omission of auxiliary labels, pharmacy contact information or practitioner ID is not to be considered a mistake.

Use your answer sheet to record your answers. You have a total of **5 prescriptions** in this station.

<u>Station Reference:</u> CPS – Compendium of Pharmaceuticals and Specialties

<u>You have 7 minutes to complete this station</u>

Written Rx 1

```
Rx 1
Patient Name: Joel Hansen
Address: 7 Montreal Avenue

                                              Correct date

    Coumadin 10 mg
    PO i tab qd x 8 weeks

    P. Venn
_____        Assume signature is correct
    P. Venn M.D.
```

Dispensed Rx 1 label

```
Rx 1                              Dr. P. Venn
Joel Hansen
                                  Correct date


        Take one tablet orally twice a day for
        eight weeks

        Coumadin 100 mg
        56 tablets
```

Written Rx 2

> Rx 2
> Patient Name: Smith Whyte
> Address: 7676 Third Road
>
>   Correct date
>
> Lescol XL 80 mg
> PO i tablet daily in the evening for 90 days
>
> *L. Benjamin*
> _____ Assume signature is correct
> L. Benjamin M.D.

Dispensed Rx 2 label

> Rx 2   Dr. L. Benjamin
> Smith Whyte
>   Correct date
>
> Take one tablet orally once a day for 90 days
>
> Leacol XL 80 mg
> 90 tablets

Written Rx 3

Rx 3
Patient Name: Barb Williamson
Address: 66-700 Hill Street

                                                                         Correct date

Uloric 80 mg
i tab qd x 30 days for gout

O. Xavier
_____ Assume signature is correct
O. Xavier M.D.

Dispensed Rx 3 label

Rx 3   Dr. O. Xavier
Barb Williamson
                                                  Correct date

Take one tablet once a day for 30 days
for gout

Uloric 80 mg
30 tablets

Written Rx 4

```
Rx 4
Patient Name: Candice Smith
Address: 999 Ottawa Street

                                            Correct date



            Parnate 10 mg
            20 mg daily in two divided am and pm doses x 3 weeks
            for depression

        D. Thomas
    _____    Assume signature is correct
        D. Thomas M.D.
```

Dispensed Rx 4 label

```
Rx 4                                    Dr. D. Thomas
Candice Smith
                                        Correct date


        Take one tablet in the morning and one
        tablet in the evening daily for three
        weeks for depression

        Parnate 10 mg
        42 tablets
```

Written Rx 5

> Rx 5
> Patient Name: Jaden Campbell
> Address: 22 Hill Avenue
>
> Correct date
>
> Pradax 75 mg capsules
> 300 mg daily in two divided doses for 50 days
>
> *X. Kassam*
> _____ Assume signature is correct
> X. Kassam M.D.

Dispensed Rx 5 label

> Rx 5   Dr. X. Kassam
> Jaden Campbell
>   Correct date
>
> Take two capsules twice a day for
> 50 days
>
>   Pradax 75 mg
>   200 tablets

Answer Sheet: Prescription Labels Check

Rx 1	Is this prescription label consistent with the prescription? Yes No What would you correct?
Rx 2	Is this prescription label consistent with the prescription? Yes No What would you correct?
Rx 3	Is this prescription label consistent with the prescription? Yes No What would you correct?
Rx 4	Is this prescription label consistent with the prescription? Yes No What would you correct?
Rx 5	Is this prescription label consistent with the prescription? Yes No What would you correct?

Answer Key #5

Rx 1	Is this prescription label consistent with the prescription? No What would you correct? Wrong drug strength Wrong instructions
Rx 2	Is this prescription label consistent with the prescription? No What would you correct? Incomplete instructions (add: in the evening) Wrong drug name
Rx 3	Is this prescription label consistent with the prescription? Yes What would you correct?
Rx 4	Is this prescription label consistent with the prescription? Yes What would you correct?
Rx 5	Is this prescription label consistent with the prescription? Yes What would you correct?

Non Interactive Case #6: Prescription Labels Check

Candidate instructions:

Identify any mistakes, omissions or concerns on each prescription label. Assume each prescription is correct and omission of auxiliary labels, pharmacy contact information or practitioner ID is not to be considered a mistake.
Use your answer sheet to record your answers. You have a total of **3 prescriptions** in this station.
Station Reference: CPS – Compendium of Pharmaceuticals and Specialties

You have 7 minutes to complete this station

Written Rx 1

> Rx 1
> Patient Name: Veera Smith
> Address: 3 Hope Street
>
> Correct date
>
> Betagan 0.5%
> 1 drop in each eye twice a day for 7 days
>
> *K. John*
> _____ Assume signature is correct
> K. John M.D.

Dispensed Rx 1 label

> Rx 1   Dr. K. John
> Veera Smith
>   Correct date
>
> Place one drop in each eye
> twice a day for seven days
>
> Betagan 1% solution

Written Rx 2

```
Rx 2
Patient Name: Tannis Spring
Address: 34A Street

                                        Correct date


    Meridia
    10 mg tab once a day x 4 weeks


       N. Smith
    _____          Assume signature is correct
       N. Smith M.D.
```

Dispensed Rx 2 label

```
Rx 2                                    Dr. N. Smith
Tannis Spring
                                        Correct date


        Take one or two tablets once
        a day for four weeks

    Meridia 10 mg

    30 tablets
```

Written Rx 3

```
Rx 3
Patient Name: Fanny Pete
Address: 2123 Street

                                        Correct date


        Sibelium
        5 mg tab once a day x 4 weeks for headache


            F. Tom
        _____   Assume signature is correct
              F. Tom M.D.
```

Dispensed Rx 3 label

```
Rx 3                                    Dr. P. Tom
Fanny Pete
                                        Correct date


        Take one tablet once a day for four
        weeks for headache

    Sibelium 5 mg

    28 tablets
```

Answer Sheet: Prescription Labels Check

Rx 1	Is this prescription label consistent with the prescription? Yes No What would you correct?
Rx 2	Is this prescription label consistent with the prescription? Yes No What would you correct?
Rx 3	Is this prescription label consistent with the prescription? Yes No What would you correct?

Answer Key #6

Rx 1	Is this prescription label consistent with the prescription? No What would you correct? Wrong drug strength.
Rx 2	Is this prescription label consistent with the prescription? No What would you correct? Wrong dosing/instructions. Wrong number of tablets.
Rx 3	Is this prescription label consistent with the prescription? No What would you correct? Wrong physician initial.

Non Interactive Case #7: Prescription Labels Check

Candidate instructions:

Identify any mistakes, omissions or concerns on each prescription label. Assume each prescription is correct and omission of auxiliary labels, pharmacy contact information or practitioner ID is not to be considered a mistake.
Use your answer sheet to record your answers. You have a total of **3 prescriptions** in this station.
Station Reference: CPS – Compendium of Pharmaceuticals and Specialties

You have 7 minutes to complete this station

Written Rx 1

```
Rx 1
Patient Name: Veronica Sam
Address: 234th Street

                                                    Correct date

        Xenical
        120 mg cap i tid for 2 weeks


         T. June
        _____  Assume signature is correct
         T. June M.D.
```

Dispensed Rx 1 label

```
Rx 1                                    Dr. T. June
Veronica Sam
                                        Correct date

        Take one capsule three times
          a day for two weeks

        Xenical 120 mg
        42 capsules
```

Written Rx 2

```
Rx 2
Patient Name: Min Kim
Address: Heron Road

                                          Correct date


    Betaloc
    50 mg qid x 30 days



        P. Wong
    _____   Assume signature is correct
        P. Wong M.D.
```

Dispensed Rx 2 label

```
Rx 2                              Dr. P. Wong
Min Kim
                                  Correct date

        Take one tablet four times
          a day for thirty days


    Betaloc 50 mg

    120 tablets
```

Written Rx 3

```
Rx 2
Patient Name: Kiana Simon
Address: 129 Sun Drive

                                        Correct date


        Glucophage
        1500 mg daily divided tid x 3 weeks




        P. Ahmed
        _____     Assume signature is correct
           P. Ahmed M.D.
```

Dispensed Rx 3 label

```
Rx 3                              Dr. P. Ahmed
Kiana Summer
                                  Correct date

        Take one tablet three times
        a day for three weeks

    Glucophage 500 mg

    63 tablets
```

Answer Sheet: Prescription Labels Check

Rx 1	Is this prescription label consistent with the prescription? Yes No What would you correct?
Rx 2	Is this prescription label consistent with the prescription? Yes No What would you correct?
Rx 3	Is this prescription label consistent with the prescription? Yes No What would you correct?

Answer Key #7

Rx 1	Is this prescription label consistent with the prescription? Yes What would you correct?
Rx 2	Is this prescription label consistent with the prescription? Yes What would you correct?
Rx 3	Is this prescription label consistent with the prescription? No What would you correct? Incorrect patient name

Non Interactive Case #8: Prescription Labels Check

Candidate instructions:

Identify any mistakes, omissions or concerns on each prescription label. Assume each prescription is correct and omission of auxiliary labels, pharmacy contact information or practitioner ID is not to be considered a mistake.
Use your answer sheet to record your answers. You have a total of **3 prescriptions** in this station.
Station Reference: CPS – Compendium of Pharmaceuticals and Specialties

You have 7 minutes to complete this station

Written Rx 1

```
Rx 1
Patient Name: Kim Spring
Address: 12 Skye Avenue

                                          Correct date

    GlucoNorm
    PO 2 mg once a day x 6 weeks

      N. Ali
    _____    Assume signature is correct
      N. Ali M.D.
```

Dispensed Rx 1 label

```
Rx 1                              Dr. N. Wang
Kim Spring
                                  Correct date

        Take one tablet once
         a day for six weeks

    GlucoDerm 2 mg

    42 tablets
```

302

Written Rx 2

```
Rx 1
Patient Name: Bob Murphy
Address: 56 3rd Avenue

                                          Correct date


    Ampicillin
    250 mg q6h x 7 days



        J. Young
    _____  Assume signature is correct
        J. Young M.D.
```

Dispensed Rx 2 label

```
Rx 2                                      Dr. J. Young
Bob Murphy
                                          Correct date

            Take one tablet every
            six hours for 7 days

        Ampicillin 250 mg

        27 tablets
```

Written Rx 3

```
Rx 3
Patient Name: Meena Singh
Address: 33 Angel Street

                                           Correct date


        Tylenol #3
        1 tablet q12h for pain
        Mitte: 15 tablets



           G. Ryan
        _____      Assume signature is correct
           G. Ryan M.D.
```

Dispensed Rx 3 label

```
Rx 3                                Dr. G. Ryan
Meena Singh
                                    Correct date

             Take one tablet every
             twelve hours for pain


        Tylenol #3

        15 tablets
```

Answer Sheet: Prescription Labels Check

Rx 1	Is this prescription label consistent with the prescription? Yes No What would you correct?
Rx 2	Is this prescription label consistent with the prescription? Yes No What would you correct?
Rx 3	Is this prescription label consistent with the prescription? Yes No What would you correct?

Answer Key #8

Rx 1	Is this prescription label consistent with the prescription? No What would you correct? Wrong physician name. Wrong drug name.
Rx 2	Is this prescription label consistent with the prescription? No What would you correct? Wrong number of tablets (28 tablets)
Rx 3	Is this prescription label consistent with the prescription? Yes What would you correct?

Non Interactive Case #9: Prescription Labels Check

Candidate instructions:

Identify any mistakes, omissions or concerns on each prescription label. Assume each prescription is correct and omission of auxiliary labels, pharmacy contact information or practitioner ID is not to be considered a mistake.

Use your answer sheet to record your answers. You have a total of **3 prescriptions** in this station.

Station Reference: CPS – Compendium of Pharmaceuticals and Specialties

You have 7 minutes to complete this station

Written Rx 1

```
Rx 1
Patient Name: Amanda Jim
Address: 214A Street

                                          Correct date

   Nexium
   40 mg once a day for GERD
   Mitte: 5 weeks

      H. June
   _____   Assume signature is correct
      H. June M.D.
```

Dispensed Rx 1 label

```
Rx 1                              Dr. H. June
Amanda Jim
                                  Correct date

        Take two tablets once a day
          for GERD for five weeks

     Nexium 20 mg
     70 tablets
```

Written Rx 2

```
Rx 2
Patient Name: Gurpreet Gill
Address: 3 Summer Road

                                    Correct date


Bezalip SR
400 mg once a day
Mitte: 60 tablets



      T. Thomas
_____    Assume signature is correct
      T. Thomas M.D.
```

Dispensed Rx 2 label

```
Rx 2                                 Dr. T. Thomas
Gurpreet Gill
                                     Correct date

          Take one tablet once a week

          Bezalip SR 400 mg

          60 tablets
```

Written Rx 3

```
Rx 3
Patient Name: Mary Paul
Address: 334 - 5th Avenue

                                                    Correct date


    Sporanox
    100 mg cap once a day for oral candidiasis
    Mitte: 2 weeks



        T. Thomas
    _____   Assume signature is correct
        T. Thomas M.D.
```

Dispensed Rx 3 label

```
Rx 3                                    Dr. T. Thomas
Mary Paul
                                        Correct date


        Take one capsule once a
        day for oral candidiasis
        for three weeks

    Sporanox 100 mg

    14 tablets
```

Answer Sheet: Prescription Labels Check

Rx 1	Is this prescription label consistent with the prescription? Yes No What would you correct?
Rx 2	Is this prescription label consistent with the prescription? Yes No What would you correct?
Rx 3	Is this prescription label consistent with the prescription? Yes No What would you correct?

Answer Key #9

Rx 1	Is this prescription label consistent with the prescription? Yes What would you correct?
Rx 2	Is this prescription label consistent with the prescription? No What would you correct? Wrong dosing/instructions.
Rx 3	Is this prescription label consistent with the prescription? No What would you correct? Wrong duration of treatment.

Non Interactive Case #10: Prescription Labels Check

Candidate instructions:

Identify any mistakes, omissions or concerns on each prescription label. Assume each prescription is correct and omission of auxiliary labels, pharmacy contact information or practitioner ID is not to be considered a mistake.
Use your answer sheet to record your answers. You have a total of **3 prescriptions** in this station.
Station Reference: CPS – Compendium of Pharmaceuticals and Specialties

You have 7 minutes to complete this station

Written Rx 1

```
Rx 1
Patient Name: Von Smith
Address: 21A Street

                                        Correct date

       Accuretic
       20/25 tab i qid x 3 weeks

         N. Jim
       _____   Assume signature is correct
            N. Jimmon M.D.
```

Dispensed Rx 1 label

```
Rx 1                              Dr. N. Jemon
Von Smith
                                  Correct date

         Take one tablet four times
         a day for three weeks

         Accuretic 20/25
         84 tablets
```

Written Rx 2

```
Rx 2
Patient Name: Wayne Park
Address: 211 3rd Avenue

                                          Correct date


        Accolate
        20 mg bid for asthma
        Mitte: 60 days



        N. Lam
        _____  Assume signature is correct
        N. Lam M.D.
```

Dispensed Rx 2 label

```
Rx 2                            Dr. N. Lam
Wayne Park
                                Correct date

            Take one tablet once a
            day for sixty days

        Accolate 20 mg

        60 tablets
```

Written Rx 3

```
Rx 3
Patient Name: Liam Scott
Address: 12 Little Street

                                            Correct date


Zovirax
400 mg tid for genital herpes
Mitte: 10 days



       R. Kassam
_____      Assume signature is correct
      R. Kassam M.D.
```

Dispensed Rx 3 label

```
Rx 3                                      Dr. R. Kassam
Liam Scott
                                          Correct date

         Take one tablet three times
         a day for ten days

      Zovirax 400 mg

      30 tablets
```

Answer Sheet: Prescription Labels Check

Rx 1	Is this prescription label consistent with the prescription? Yes　　　　　　No What would you correct?
Rx 2	Is this prescription label consistent with the prescription? Yes　　　　　　No What would you correct?
Rx 3	Is this prescription label consistent with the prescription? Yes　　　　　　No What would you correct?

Answer Key #10

Rx 1	Is this prescription label consistent with the prescription? No What would you correct? Physician name spelled wrong.
Rx 2	Is this prescription label consistent with the prescription? No What would you correct? Wrong dosing. Wrong number of tablets.
Rx 3	Is this prescription label consistent with the prescription? Yes What would you correct?

Non Interactive Case #11: Prescription Labels Check

Candidate instructions:

Identify any mistakes, omissions or concerns on each prescription label. Assume each prescription is correct and omission of auxiliary labels, pharmacy contact information or practitioner ID is not to be considered a mistake.
Use your answer sheet to record your answers. You have a total of **3 prescriptions** in this station.
Station Reference: CPS – Compendium of Pharmaceuticals and Specialties

You have 7 minutes to complete this station

Written Rx 1

```
Rx 1
Patient Name: Cathy Fong
Address: 21 2nd street

                                                    Correct date


        Efavirenz
        600 mg daily x 90 days

          H. Kong
    _____  Assume signature is correct
          H. Kong M.D.
```

Dispensed Rx 1 label

```
Rx 1                                    Dr. H. Kong
Cathy Fong
                                        Correct date

            Take one tablet daily for 90 days

            Efavirenz 600 mg
            90 tablets
```

Written Rx 2

```
Rx 2
Patient Name: Kim Don
Address: 21 Green Street

                                    Correct date


Captopril
50 mg tid x 2 weeks




      A. Hammond
_____     Assume signature is correct
      A.  Hammond M.D.
```

Dispensed Rx 2 label

```
Rx 2                          Dr. A. Hammond
Kim Don
                              Correct date


        Take two tablets three times
        a day for two weeks


        Captopril 25 mg

        78 tablets
```

Written Rx 3

```
Rx 3
Patient Name: Karyn Cains
Address:  Moose Street

                                        Correct date


      Coumadin
      10 mg daily
      Mitte: 30 tablets



        L. Singh
    _____   Assume signature is correct
        L. Singh M.D.
```

Dispensed Rx 3 label

```
Rx 3                                    Dr. L. Singh
Kareen Cains
                                        Correct date


        Take one tablet daily for thirty days

        Coumadin 10 mg

        30 tablets
```

Answer Sheet: Prescription Labels Check

Rx 1	Is this prescription label consistent with the prescription? Yes No What would you correct?
Rx 2	Is this prescription label consistent with the prescription? Yes No What would you correct?
Rx 3	Is this prescription label consistent with the prescription? Yes No What would you correct?

Answer Key #11

Rx 1	Is this prescription label consistent with the prescription? Yes What would you correct?
Rx 2	Is this prescription label consistent with the prescription? No What would you correct? Wrong number of tablets (84 tablets)
Rx 3	Is this prescription label consistent with the prescription? No What would you correct? Patient name spelled wrong.

Non Interactive Case #12: Prescription Labels Check

Candidate instructions:

Identify any mistakes, omissions or concerns on each prescription label. Assume each prescription is correct and omission of auxiliary labels, pharmacy contact information or practitioner ID is not to be considered a mistake.
Use your answer sheet to record your answers. You have a total of **3 prescriptions** in this station.
Station Reference: CPS – Compendium of Pharmaceuticals and Specialties

You have 7 minutes to complete this station

Written Rx 1

```
Rx 1
Patient Name: Pamela Park
Address: 341 Edmonton Street

                                            Correct date


        Furosemide
        80 mg divided bid x 5 weeks

        G. Norm
                                    Assume signature is correct
        _____
        G. Norm M.D.
```

Dispensed Rx 1 label

```
Rx 1                            Dr. G. Norm
Pamela Park
                                Correct date


        Take one tablet twice a
        day for five weeks

        Furosemide 40 mg

        70 tablets
```

Written Rx 2

```
Rx 2
Patient Name: Nancy Simms
Address: 23 3rd Street

                                        Correct date


       Halcion
       0.5 mg once a day
       Mitte: 2 weeks



         D. Paul
    _____       Assume signature is correct
       D. Paul M.D.
```

Dispensed Rx 2 label

```
Rx 2                              Dr. D. Paul
Nancy Simms
                                  Correct date


         Take two tablets once a
         day for two weeks

    Halsin 0.25 mg

    28 tablets
```

Written Rx 3

```
Rx 3
Patient Name: Don Reid
Address: 2 Winter Avenue

                                          Correct date


       Azithromycin
       500 mg q24h x 5 days




         R. Lee
    _____       Assume signature is correct
         R. Lee M.D.
```

Dispensed Rx 3 label

```
Rx 3                              Dr. R. Lee
Don Reid
                                  Correct date


       Take one tablet every 24 hours
              for five days

       Azithromycin 500 mg

          5 tablets
```

Answer Sheet: Prescription Labels Check

Rx 1	Is this prescription label consistent with the prescription? Yes No What would you correct?
Rx 2	Is this prescription label consistent with the prescription? Yes No What would you correct?
Rx 3	Is this prescription label consistent with the prescription? Yes No What would you correct?

Answer Key #12

Rx 1	Is this prescription label consistent with the prescription? Yes What would you correct?
Rx 2	Is this prescription label consistent with the prescription? No What would you correct? Wrong drug name.
Rx 3	Is this prescription label consistent with the prescription? Yes What would you correct?

Non Interactive Case #13: Prescription Labels Check

Candidate instructions:

Identify any mistakes, omissions or concerns on each prescription label. Assume each prescription is correct and omission of auxiliary labels, pharmacy contact information or practitioner ID is not to be considered a mistake.
Use your answer sheet to record your answers. You have a total of **4 prescriptions** in this station.
Station Reference: CPS – Compendium of Pharmaceuticals and Specialties

You have 7 minutes to complete this station

Written Rx 1

```
Rx 1
Patient Name: Miranda Smith
Address: 35 Hill Street

                                              Correct date


        Gleevec
        800 mg divided bid for leukemia for 90 days

            K. Junior
        _____   Assume signature is correct
            K. Junior M.D.
```

Dispensed Rx 1 label

```
Rx 1                                    Dr. K. June
Miranda Smith
                                        Correct date


        Take one tablet twice a day for
        leukemia for 90 days

           Glovec 400 mg
           180 tablets
```

Written Rx 2

Rx 2
Patient Name: Heather Moon
Address: 34C Street

                                                                                  Correct date

Fluconazole
150 mg po x 1 dose for vaginal candidiasis

N. Smith
_____ Assume signature is correct
N. Smith M.D.

Dispensed Rx 2 label

Rx 2   Dr. N. Smith
Heather Moon
                                                          Correct date

                    Take three tablets once
                     for vaginal candidiasis

Fluconazole 50 mg

3 tablets

Written Rx 3

Rx 3
Patient Name: Fanny May
Address: 2123 Street

Correct date

Mirtazapine
15 mg tab once a day x 8 weeks

F. Tom
_____ Assume signature is correct
F. Tom M.D.

Dispensed Rx 3 label

Rx 3   Dr. P. Tom
Fanny Pete
                                        Correct date

Take one tablet once a day
for eight weeks

Mirtazapine 15 mg

56 tablets

Written Rx 4

```
Rx 4
Patient Name: Lynn Ryan
Address: 311 Summer Street

                                        Correct date


Norfloxacin
400 mg po bid 1 h ac x 3 days



    K. Lam
_____       Assume signature is correct
    K. Lam M.D.
```

Dispensed Rx 4 label

```
Rx 4                          Dr. K. Liam
Lynna Ryan
                              Correct date


    Take one tablet twice a day one hour
    after a meal for three days


Norfloxacin 400 mg

6 tablets
```

Answer Sheet: Prescription Labels Check

Rx 1	Is this prescription label consistent with the prescription? Yes No What would you correct?
Rx 2	Is this prescription label consistent with the prescription? Yes No What would you correct?
Rx 3	Is this prescription label consistent with the prescription? Yes No What would you correct?
Rx 4	Is this prescription label consistent with the prescription? Yes No What would you correct?

Answer Key #13

Rx 1	Is this prescription label consistent with the prescription? No What would you correct? Wrong drug name. Wrong physician name
Rx 2	Is this prescription label consistent with the prescription? Yes What would you correct?
Rx 3	Is this prescription label consistent with the prescription? No What would you correct? Wrong patient's name. Wrong physician's name.
Rx 4	Is this prescription label consistent with the prescription? No What would you correct? Wrong dosing. Wrong patient's name Wrong physician's name

Non Interactive Case #14: Prescription Labels Check

Candidate instructions:

Identify any mistakes, omissions or concerns on each prescription label. Assume each prescription is correct and omission of auxiliary labels, pharmacy contact information or practitioner ID is not to be considered a mistake.

Use your answer sheet to record your answers. You have a total of **4 prescriptions** in this station.

Station Reference: CPS – Compendium of Pharmaceuticals and Specialties

You have 7 minutes to complete this station

Written Rx 1

```
Rx 1
Patient Name: Kim Park
Address: 30 Seaview Drive

                                               Correct date


        Neomycin 3.5 mg/g cream
        Apply twice a day x 7 days to affected area


         K. Gill
        _____  Assume signature is correct
         K. Gill M.D.
```

Dispensed Rx 1 label

```
Rx 1                              Dr. K. Gill
Kim Park
                                  Correct date


         Apply twice day for seven days to
         affected area

         Neomycin 3.5 mg/ml cream
```

Written Rx 2

Rx 2
Patient Name: Timmy Hamed
Address: 22 Sunny Place

Correct date

Paliperidone
6 mg daily x 5 days, then 12 mg daily x 2 weeks

Y. Patrick
_____ Assume signature is correct
Y. Patrick M.D.

Dispensed Rx 2 label

Rx 2   Dr. Y. Patrick
Timmy Hamed
                                               Correct date

Take two tablets once a day
for five days then take fours tablets for
fourteen days

Paliperidone 3mg

66 tablets

Written Rx 3

Rx 3
Patient Name: April Lee
Address: 21 Winter Blv

                                                      Correct date

Medroxyprogesterone
20 mg tid x 4 weeks

A. Whyth
_____ Assume signature is correct
A. Whyth M.D.

Dispensed Rx 3 label

Rx 3   Dr. A. Whyth
April Lee

                                          Correct date

Take two tablets three times a day
for four weeks

Medraprogesterone 10 mg

168 tablets

Written Rx 4

Rx 4
Patient Name: Andrea Fynn
Address: 34A Street

                                                                Correct date

Norethindrone
10 mg on day 5 through day 25 of menstrual cycle for amenorrhea

N. Smith
_____ Assume signature is correct
N. Smith M.D.

Dispensed Rx 4 label

Rx 4   Dr. N. Smith
Andrea Fynn
                                      Correct date

Take two tablets on day 5 through day 25 of menstrual cycle for amenorrhea

Northrindone 10 mg

40 tablets

Answer Sheet: Prescription Labels Check

Rx 1	Is this prescription label consistent with the prescription? Yes No What would you correct?
Rx 2	Is this prescription label consistent with the prescription? Yes No What would you correct?
Rx 3	Is this prescription label consistent with the prescription? Yes No What would you correct?
Rx 4	Is this prescription label consistent with the prescription? Yes No What would you correct?

Answer Key #14

Rx 1	Is this prescription label consistent with the prescription? No What would you correct? Wrong drug formulation.
Rx 2	Is this prescription label consistent with the prescription? Yes What would you correct?
Rx 3	Is this prescription label consistent with the prescription? No What would you correct? Wrong drug name.
Rx 4	Is this prescription label consistent with the prescription? No What would you correct? Wrong drug name. Wrong drug strength.

Non Interactive Case #15: Prescription Labels Check

Candidate instructions:

Identify any mistakes, omissions or concerns on each prescription label. Assume each prescription is correct and omission of auxiliary labels, pharmacy contact information or practitioner ID is not to be considered a mistake.
Use your answer sheet to record your answers. You have a total of **4 prescriptions** in this station.
Station Reference: CPS – Compendium of Pharmaceuticals and Specialties

You have 7 minutes to complete this station

Written Rx 1

```
Rx 1
Patient Name: Mary Smith
Address: 398 Hope Drive

                                          Correct date


      Megestrol 40 mg/ml
      Take 5 ml q6h x 21 days to enhance appetite


        G. John
    _____    Assume signature is correct
         G. John M.D.
```

Dispensed Rx 1 label

```
Rx 1                                      Dr. G. John
Mary Smith
                                          Correct date


        Take five milliliters every six hours
          for twenty one days to enhance appetite

        Megestrol 40 mg
```

339

Written Rx 2

Rx 2
Patient Name: Jake Min
Address: 340 2nd Street

                                                                  Correct date

Meloxicam 7.5 mg
2 tabs once a day x 6 weeks

T. Fall
_____ Assume signature is correct
T. Fall M.D.

Dispensed Rx 2 label

Rx 2   Dr. T. Fall
Jaky Min

                                     Correct date

Take two tablets once
a day for five weeks

Meloxicam 7.5 mg

84 tablets

Written Rx 3

Rx 3
Patient Name: Nancy Peter
Address: 2123 Street

Correct date

Granisetron
3.1mg patch q5days for 10 days for nausea

B. Ali
_____ Assume signature is correct
B. Ali M.D.

Dispensed Rx 3 label

Rx 3 Dr. B. Ali
Nancy Peter
Correct date

Take one tablet every five days
for ten days for nausea

Granisetron 3.1mg

2 patches

Written Rx 4

Rx 4
Patient Name: Rick Johnson
Address: 2123 Street

                                                      Correct date

Linezolid 100 mg/5ml susp
300 mg q12h x 14 days for skin infection

F. Koo
_____   Assume signature is correct
F. Koo M.D.

Dispensed Rx 4 label

Rx 4   Dr. F. Koo
Rick Johnson
                                        Correct date

Take one tablespoon every twelve hours
for fourteen days for skin infection

Linezolid 100 mg/ 5ml suspension

Answer Sheet: Prescription Labels Check

Rx 1	Is this prescription label consistent with the prescription? Yes　　　　　　　No What would you correct?
Rx 2	Is this prescription label consistent with the prescription? Yes　　　　　　　No What would you correct?
Rx 3	Is this prescription label consistent with the prescription? Yes　　　　　　　No What would you correct?
Rx 4	Is this prescription label consistent with the prescription? Yes　　　　　　　No What would you correct?

Answer Key #15

Rx 1	Is this prescription label consistent with the prescription? No What would you correct? Wrong drug formulation.
Rx 2	Is this prescription label consistent with the prescription? No What would you correct? Wrong duration of treatment. Wrong patient's name.
Rx 3	Is this prescription label consistent with the prescription? No What would you correct? Wrong administration route
Rx 4	Is this prescription label consistent with the prescription? Yes What would you correct?

Non Interactive Case #16: Prescription Labels Check

Candidate instructions:

Identify any mistakes, omissions or concerns on each prescription label. Assume each prescription is correct and omission of auxiliary labels, pharmacy contact information or practitioner ID is not to be considered a mistake.

Use your answer sheet to record your answers. You have a total of **4 prescriptions** in this station.

Station Reference: CPS – Compendium of Pharmaceuticals and Specialties

You have 7 minutes to complete this station

Written Rx 1

> Rx 1
> Patient Name: Lory Sunny
> Address: 344 Eagle Street
>
> Correct date
>
> Acitretin
> 25 mg cap po once a day x 7 days
>
> *K. John*
> _____ Assume signature is correct
> K. John M.D.

Dispensed Rx 1 label

> Rx 1   Dr. K. John
> Lory Sunny
>
> Take one capsule daily for seven days
>
> Bacitretin 25 mg
> 7 tablets

Written Rx 2

```
Rx 2
Patient Name: Pamela Malik
Address: 34A Rain Court

                                    Correct date


       Amitriptyline
       50 mg once a day for 8 weeks




         N. Smith
       _____   Assume signature is correct
         N. Smith M.D.
```

Dispensed Rx 2 label

```
Rx 2                              Dr. N. Smith
Pamela Malik
                                  Correct date


        Take one tablet once
        a day for eight weeks

     Amitriptyline 25mg

     110 tablets
```

Written Rx 3

```
Rx 3
Patient Name: Frank Paul
Address: 55-2nd Street

                                            Correct date


        Atovaquone 750 mg/ 5ml
        5 ml bid for 21 days




        F. Bryan
        _____      Assume signature is correct
           F. Bryan M.D.
```

Dispensed Rx 3 label

```
Rx 3                                  Dr. F. Bryan
Frank Paul
                                      Correct date


        Take one tablepoon twice a day
        for twenty one days


        Atovaquone 75 mg/ 5ml suspension
```

Written Rx 4

Rx 4
Patient Name: Veera Smith
Address: 3 Hope Street

                                                                           Correct date

Glycopyrrolate
2 mg tid x 1wk then decrease to 1 mg bid x 4wks for peptic ulcer

K. John
_____ Assume signature is correct
K. John M.D.

Dispensed Rx 4 label

Rx 4   Dr. K. John
Veera Smith
                                                Correct date

Take two tablets three times a day for
one week then take one tablet twice a day
for four weeks for peptic ulcer

Glycopyrrolate 1 mg

98 tablets

Answer Sheet: Prescription Labels Check

Rx 1	Is this prescription label consistent with the prescription? Yes　　　　　　　No What would you correct?
Rx 2	Is this prescription label consistent with the prescription? Yes　　　　　　　No What would you correct?
Rx 3	Is this prescription label consistent with the prescription? Yes　　　　　　　No What would you correct?
Rx 4	Is this prescription label consistent with the prescription? Yes　　　　　　　No What would you correct?

Answer Key #16

Rx 1	Is this prescription label consistent with the prescription? No What would you correct? Wrong drug name. Missing date.
Rx 2	Is this prescription label consistent with the prescription? No What would you correct? Wrong dosing. Wrong number of tablets.
Rx 3	Is this prescription label consistent with the prescription? No What would you correct? Wrong drug strength. Wrong dosing.
Rx 4	Is this prescription label consistent with the prescription? Yes What would you correct?

Non Interactive Case #17: Prescription Labels Check

Candidate instructions:

Identify any mistakes, omissions or concerns on each prescription label. Assume each prescription is correct and omission of auxiliary labels, pharmacy contact information or practitioner ID is not to be considered a mistake.

Use your answer sheet to record your answers. You have a total of **4 prescriptions** in this station.

Station Reference: CPS – Compendium of Pharmaceuticals and Specialties

You have 7 minutes to complete this station

Written Rx 1

```
Rx 1
Patient Name: Marie Simon
Address: 3 Marmot Road

                                              Correct date

       Atorvastatin
       Start at 10mg daily, increase by 10 mg every 2 weeks up to 50 mg
       daily then continue at 50 mg daily for 4 weeks

         P. Wang
       _____  Assume signature is correct
            P. Wang M.D.
```

Dispensed Rx 1 label

```
Rx 1                                          Dr. K. Wang
Marie Simon
                                              Correct date

              Take one tablet daily for two weeks
              Then two tablets for two more weeks
              Then 3 tablets for two more weeks
              Then 4 tablets for two more weeks
              Then 5 tablets for four more weeks

       Atorvastatin 10 mg
       282 tablets
```

Written Rx 2

Rx 2
Patient Name: Renee Wayne
Address: 34 Major Road

                                                               Correct date

Nevirapine
200 mg once a day x 14 days
then increase to 200 mg bid x 4 weeks

W. Arthur
_____   Assume signature is correct
W. Arthur M.D.

Dispensed Rx 2 label

Rx 2   Dr. N. Smith
Renee White
                                            Correct date

Take two tablets once a day for 14 days
Then take one tablet twice a day for four weeks

Nebirapine 200mg

70 tablets

Written Rx 3

```
Rx 3
Patient Name: Fanny Koo
Address: 2123 Street

                                              Correct date


       Nifedipine
       20 mg cap tid x 3 weeks for angina




         F. Thomas
       _____  Assume signature is correct
            F. Thomas M.D.
```

Dispensed Rx 3 label

```
Rx 3                                   Dr. F. Thomas
Fanny Koo
                                       Correct date

         Take one capsule three times a day
             for three weeks for angina


         Nifedipine 20 mg

         63 tablets
```

Written Rx 4

```
Rx 4
Patient Name: Tannis John
Address: 34A Street

                                    Correct date


        Prednisolone
        5 mg tab bid cc x 30 days



           Y. Smith
        _____     Assume signature is correct
           Y. Smith M.D.
```

Dispensed Rx 4 label

```
Rx 4                              Dr. Y. Smith
Tannis John


         Take one tablet twice a day for 30 days


       Prednisolone 5 mg

       60 tablets
```

<u>Answer Sheet</u>: Prescription Labels Check

Rx 1	Is this prescription label consistent with the prescription? Yes No What would you correct?
Rx 2	Is this prescription label consistent with the prescription? Yes No What would you correct?
Rx 3	Is this prescription label consistent with the prescription? Yes No What would you correct?
Rx 4	Is this prescription label consistent with the prescription? Yes No What would you correct?

Answer Key #17

Rx 1	Is this prescription label consistent with the prescription? No What would you correct? Wrong physician's name. Wrong number of tablets. Liver function monitoring after 6 to 12 weeks of therapy
Rx 2	Is this prescription label consistent with the prescription? No What would you correct? Wrong dosing. Wrong drug name.
Rx 3	Is this prescription label consistent with the prescription? Yes What would you correct?
Rx 4	Is this prescription label consistent with the prescription? No What would you correct? Incomplete dosing. Add with meals (cc) Missing date.

Non Interactive Case #18: Prescription Labels Check

Candidate instructions:

Identify any mistakes, omissions or concerns on each prescription label. Assume each prescription is correct and omission of auxiliary labels, pharmacy contact information or practitioner ID is not to be considered a mistake.

Use your answer sheet to record your answers. You have a total of **4 prescriptions** in this station.

Station Reference: CPS – Compendium of Pharmaceuticals and Specialties

You have 7 minutes to complete this station

Written Rx 1

```
Rx 1
Patient Name: Art Smith
Address: 300 Hope Road

                                                    Correct date


      Atorvastatin
      40 mg daily x 6weeks


         K, John
_____  Assume signature is correct
        K. John M.D.
```

Dispensed Rx 1 label

```
Rx 1                                      Dr. K. John
Art Smith


            Take two tablets once a day
                  for six weeks

         Atorvastatin 20 mg
         84 tablets
```

Written Rx 2

```
Rx 2
Patient Name: Linda Shims
Address: 355A Street

                                           Correct date


        Oxacillin 250 mg/5 ml
        500 mg q4h x 10 days



           N. Joy
        _____    Assume signature is correct
           N. Joy M.D.
```

Dispensed Rx 2 label

```
Rx 2                           Dr. N. Joy
Linda Shims
                               Correct date

        Take two tablespoons every four hours
        for ten days

        Oxacillin 250 mg/ ml
```

Written Rx 3

> Rx 3
> Patient Name: Tim Low
> Address: 21B Street
>
> Correct date
>
> Mesalamine 500 mg
> 1 supp pr bid x 6 weeks for ulcerative colitis
>
> *F. Kassam*
> _____ Assume signature is correct
> F. Kassam M.D.

Dispensed Rx 3 label

> Rx 3   Dr. F. Kassam
> Tim Low
>   Correct date
>
>   Take one tablet twice a day
>   for six weeks
>
>   Mesamine 500 mg
>
>   84 tablets

Written Rx 4

```
Rx 4
Patient Name: Jamie Scott
Address: 212 Vancouver Street

                                          Correct date


         Methylphenidate SR
         20 mg once a day before breakfast for 2 wks for ADD



             P. Thomas
         _____       Assume signature is correct
            P. Thomas M.D.
```

Dispensed Rx 4 label

```
Rx 4                                    Dr. P. Thomas
Jamie Scott
                                        Correct date

     Take one tablet once a day before breakfast
     for two weeks for Attention Deficit Disorder

     Methylphenidate 20 mg

     14 tablets
```

Answer Sheet: Prescription Labels Check

Rx 1	Is this prescription label consistent with the prescription? Yes　　　　　　　No What would you correct?
Rx 2	Is this prescription label consistent with the prescription? Yes　　　　　　　No What would you correct?
Rx 3	Is this prescription label consistent with the prescription? Yes　　　　　　　No What would you correct?
Rx 4	Is this prescription label consistent with the prescription? Yes　　　　　　　No What would you correct?

Answer Key #18

Rx 1	Is this prescription label consistent with the prescription? No What would you correct? Missing date
Rx 2	Is this prescription label consistent with the prescription? No What would you correct? Wrong dosing. Wrong drug strength.
Rx 3	Is this prescription label consistent with the prescription? No What would you correct? Wrong administration route. Wrong drug name.
Rx 4	Is this prescription label consistent with the prescription? No What would you correct? Wrong drug formulation. Add SR

Non Interactive Case #19: Prescription Labels Check

Candidate instructions:

Identify any mistakes, omissions or concerns on each prescription label. Assume each prescription is correct and omission of auxiliary labels, pharmacy contact information or practitioner ID is not to be considered a mistake.
Use your answer sheet to record your answers. You have a total of **5 prescriptions** in this station.
Station Reference: CPS – Compendium of Pharmaceuticals and Specialties

You have 7 minutes to complete this station

Written Rx 1

Rx 1
Patient Name: Veronica Smith
Address: 3 Hope Street

Correct date

Meloxicam
15 mg once a day x 8 weeks for RA

T. Young

_____ Assume signature is correct
T. Young M.D.

Dispensed Rx 1 label

Rx 1   Dr. T. Young
Veronica Smith
                                           Correct date

Take one tablet once a day for eight
weeks for rheumatoid arthritis

Meloxicam 7.5 mg
56 tablets

Written Rx 2

```
Rx 2
Patient Name: Pamela Moon
Address: 388A Sunny Road

                                          Correct date


        Mefloquine
        250 mg once/wk x 4 wks
        Then 250 mg every other wk x 10 wks



           N. Smith
        _____   Assume signature is correct
           N. Smith M.D.
```

Dispensed Rx 2 label

```
Rx 2                              Dr. N. Smith
Pamela Moon
                                  Correct date

        Take one tablet once each week for four
        weeks then one tablet every other week
        for ten weeks

        Melfaquine 250 mg

        9 tablets
```

Written Rx 3

```
Rx 3
Patient Name: Jimmy Pete
Address: 21st Street

                                        Correct date


        Flavoxate
        100 mg po tid x 30 days for incontinence




          F. Smith
        _____    Assume signature is correct
          F. Smith M.D.
```

Dispensed Rx 3 label

```
Rx 3                              Dr. F. Smith
Janny Pete
                                  Correct date

        Take one tablet three times a day
          for 30 days for incontinence

    Flavoxate 100g

       90 tablets
```

Written Rx 4

```
Rx 4
Patient Name: Halim Parker
Address: 34C Seaview Court

                                           Correct date


   Sulfamethoxazole/Trimethoprim 200 mg SMX/40 mg TMP/ 5ml
   Equivalent child dose of adult 800 mg SMX/160 mg TMP q12h x
   7 days for infection assuming a child BSA of 0.75 m²



       𝒩. Smith
   _____   Assume signature is correct
         N. Smith M.D.
```

Dispensed Rx 4 label

```
Rx 4                                    Dr. N. Sam
Halim Parker
                                        Correct date


          Take 7.5 ml every twelve hours
            for seven days for infection


             Sulfamethoxazole/Trimethoprim
          200 mg SMX/40 mg TMP/ 5ml suspension
```

Written Rx 5

> Rx 5
> Patient Name: Rory May
> Address: 21 Calgary Avenue
>
> Correct date
>
> Sulfadiazine 500mg tabs
> 150 mg/kg/day divided in 4 doses (4g/day max) for 5 days
> Child weight is 30 kg
>
> *F. Wang*
> _____ Assume signature is correct
> F. Wang M.D.

Dispensed Rx 5 label

> Rx 5   Dr. F.Wang
> Rory May
>   Correct date
>
>   Take two tablets four times a day
>   for five days
>
>   Sulfadiazine 500mg
>
>   40 tablets

Answer Sheet: Prescription Labels Check

Rx 1	Is this prescription label consistent with the prescription? Yes No What would you correct?
Rx 2	Is this prescription label consistent with the prescription? Yes No What would you correct?
Rx 3	Is this prescription label consistent with the prescription? Yes No What would you correct?
Rx 4	Is this prescription label consistent with the prescription? Yes No What would you correct?
Rx 5	Is this prescription label consistent with the prescription? Yes No What would you correct?

Answer Key #19

Rx 1	Is this prescription label consistent with the prescription? No What would you correct? Wrong drug strength.
Rx 2	Is this prescription label consistent with the prescription? No What would you correct? Wrong drug name.
Rx 3	Is this prescription label consistent with the prescription? No What would you correct? Wrong patient's name. Wrong drug strength.
Rx 4	Is this prescription label consistent with the prescription? No What would you correct? Wrong dosing. Wrong physician's name Dose (child) = [BSA (child) / BSA (adult)] x Dose (adult) BSA (adult) = 1.73 m^2 Correct dose is 8.6 ml
Rx 5	Is this prescription label consistent with the prescription? Yes What would you correct?

Non Interactive Case #20: Prescription Labels Check

Candidate instructions:

Identify any mistakes, omissions or concerns on each prescription label. Assume each prescription is correct and omission of auxiliary labels, pharmacy contact information or practitioner ID is not to be considered a mistake.
Use your answer sheet to record your answers. You have a total of **5 prescriptions** in this station.
Station Reference: CPS – Compendium of Pharmaceuticals and Specialties

You have 7 minutes to complete this station

Written Rx 1

```
Rx 1
Patient Name: Veronique George
Address: 311 Hope Street

                                              Correct date

      Timolol 0.25% sol
      1 drp od bid x 7 days


         K. Lee
      _____        Assume signature is correct
         K. Lee M.D.
```

Dispensed Rx 1 label

```
Rx 1                             Dr. K. Lee
Veronique George
                                 Correct date

         Place one drop in each eye
         twice a day for seven days

         Timolol 0.25% gel
```

370

Written Rx 2

```
Rx 2
Patient Name: Marie Henry
Address: 3 Montreal Street

                                            Correct date


    Lamotrigine
    50 mg once a day x 2 wks
    Then 50 mg bid x 2 wks
    Then increase by 100 mg daily at 2 wks interval until 300 mg bid
    Then continue at 300 mg bid for 5 wks


      A. Peter
    _____  Assume signature is correct
      A. Peter M.D.
```

Dispensed Rx 2 label

```
Rx 2                                    Dr. A. Peter
Marie Henry
                                        Correct date

        Take one tablet once a day for fourteen
        days
        Then take one tablet twice a day for
        fourteen days
        Then take two tablets twice a day for
        fourteen days
        Then take three tablets twice a day for
        thirty five days

    Lamotrigine 50 mg

    308 tablets
```

Written Rx 3

Rx 3
Patient Name: Fiona Dakota
Address: 2123 3rd Road

Correct date

Methimazole
5 mg tab q8h x 6 weeks for hyperthyroidism

F. Hakim
_____   Assume signature is correct
F. Hakim M.D.

Dispensed Rx 3 label

Rx 3   Dr. F. Hakim
Fiona Dakota
                                                     Correct date

Take one tablet every eight hours
for six weeks for hyperthyroidism

Methimazole 5 mg

128 tablets

Written Rx 4

Rx 4
Patient Name: Rene Paul
Address: 35 Fox Street

                                                  Correct date

Tetracycline 125 mg/5ml susp
250 mg tid x 10 days

L. Liam
_____ Assume signature is correct
L. Liam M.D.

Dispensed Rx 4 label

Rx 4   Dr. L. Liam
Rene Paul
                                                Correct date

Take two teaspoons three times a day for ten days

Tetracycline 125mg/ml suspension

Written Rx 5

```
Rx 5
Patient Name: Roger Smith
Address: 35 Hill Street

                                        Correct date


      Meperidine HCl 50 mg/5ml syrup
      1.5 mg/kg q4h (max: 100 mg q4h) prn for pain
      Child weight is 50 kg



        K. Junior
    _____    Assume signature is correct
        K. Junior M.D.
```

Dispensed Rx 5 label

```
Rx 5                              Dr. K. Junior
Roger Smith
                                  Correct date


        Take one tablespoon every four hours as
        needed for pain


        Meperidine HCl 50 mg/5ml syrup
```

Answer Sheet: Prescription Labels Check

Rx 1	Is this prescription label consistent with the prescription? Yes No What would you correct?
Rx 2	Is this prescription label consistent with the prescription? Yes No What would you correct?
Rx 3	Is this prescription label consistent with the prescription? Yes No What would you correct?
Rx 4	Is this prescription label consistent with the prescription? Yes No What would you correct?
Rx 5	Is this prescription label consistent with the prescription? Yes No What would you correct?

Answer Key #20

Rx 1	Is this prescription label consistent with the prescription? 　　　　　No What would you correct? Wrong drug formulation. Wrong dosing.
Rx 2	Is this prescription label consistent with the prescription? 　　　　　Yes What would you correct?
Rx 3	Is this prescription label consistent with the prescription? 　　　　　No What would you correct? Wrong number of tablets; 126 tablets.
Rx 4	Is this prescription label consistent with the prescription? 　　　　　No What would you correct? Wrong drug strength.
Rx 5	Is this prescription label consistent with the prescription? 　　　　　No What would you correct? Wrong dosing. ½ tbsp = 7.5 ml instead.

Non Interactive Case #1: New Prescriptions Check

Candidate instructions:

Identify any mistakes, omissions or concerns on each new prescription. Some prescriptions have more than one problem. Omission of practitioner ID is not to be considered a mistake.
Use your answer sheet to record your answers. You have a total of **4 prescriptions** in this station.

Station Reference: CPS – Compendium of Pharmaceuticals and Specialties

You have 7 minutes to complete this station

Written Rx 1

```
Rx 1
Patient Name: Honey Smith
Address: 3545 Hillcrest Street

                                              Correct date

        Synthroid 100 mg
        100 mg qd for hypothyroidism
        Mitte: 100 tablets



            T June
        _____     Assume signature is correct
            T. June M.D.
```

Written Rx 2

```
Rx 2
Patient Name: Paul Anderson
Address: 522A Fall Street

                                          Correct date


    Valcyte 450 mg
    PO 900 mg bid x 21days for CMV retinitis



       K. Kim
    _____        Assume signature is correct
       K. Kim M.D.
```

Written Rx 3

```
Rx 3
Patient Name: Ali Karim
Address: 991 Highview Street

                                          Correct date


    Exelon
    Start with 1.5mg bid, increase by 1.5 mg bid q2wk until 6mg bid
    then continue for 4 weeks

       D. Johnson
    _____        Assume signature is correct
       D. Johnson M.D.
```

Written Rx 4

> Rx 4
> Patient Name: Mirna Hamid
> Address: 8 Chateau Place
>
> Correct date
>
> Dilantin
> PO 300 mg in 3 divided doses daily for seizures
> Mitte: 90 days
>
> _____ Assume signature is correct
> S. Samuel M.D.

Answer Sheet: New Prescriptions Check

Rx 1	Is this prescription ready to be processed and filled? Yes No What would you correct or add?
Rx 2	Is this prescription ready to be processed and filled? Yes No What would you correct or add?
Rx 3	Is this prescription ready to be processed and filled? Yes No What would you correct or add?
Rx 4	Is this prescription ready to be processed and filled? Yes No What would you correct or add?

Answer Key #1

Rx 1	Is this prescription ready to be processed and filled? No What would you correct or add? Wrong drug strength (100 ug) Add: Take ideally 1h before or 2h after breakfast. Take consistently with regard to meals.
Rx 2	Is this prescription ready to be processed and filled? Yes What would you correct or add? Add: Do not crush tablets. Take with food.
Rx 3	Is this prescription ready to be processed and filled? Yes What would you correct or add? Add: Take with food
Rx 4	Is this prescription ready to be processed and filled? No What would you correct or add? Physician signature is missing Add: Do not take within 2-3h of antacid

Non Interactive Case #2: New Prescriptions Check

Candidate instructions:

Identify any mistakes, omissions or concerns on each new prescription. Some prescriptions have more than one problem. Omission of practitioner ID is not to be considered a mistake.
Use your answer sheet to record your answers. You have a total of **4 prescriptions** in this station.

Station Reference: CPS – Compendium of Pharmaceuticals and Specialties

You have 7 minutes to complete this station

Written Rx 1

Rx 1
Patient Name: Joel Hansen
Address: 7 Montreal Avenue

                                              Correct date

Zyprexa 100 mg
PO i tab qd for psychosis
Mitte: 60 tablets

P. Venn
_____ Assume signature is correct
P. Venn M.D.

Written Rx 2

```
Rx 2
Patient Name: Smith Whyte
Address: 7676 Third Road



        Sporanox 10 mg/ml
        PO ii caps qd x 3 days for vaginal candidiasis



        L. Benjamin
    _____  Assume signature is correct
          L. Benjamin M.D.
```

Written Rx 3

```
Rx 3
Patient Name: Moon William
Address:
                                              Correct date

Actonel 35 mg
35 mg qd x 3 months for the prevention of osteoporosis


        O. Xavier
    _____  Assume signature is correct
          O. Xavier M.D.
```

Written Rx 4

> Rx 4
> Patient Name: Cookie Park
> Address: 999 Ottawa Street
>
>   Correct date
>
> Risperdal 3 mg
> One tablet bid x 90 days for high blood pressure
>
>
>   *D. Thomas*
> _____ Assume signature is correct
>   D. Thomas M.D.

Answer Sheet: New Prescriptions Check

Rx 1	Is this prescription ready to be processed and filled? Yes No What would you correct or add?
Rx 2	Is this prescription ready to be processed and filled? Yes No What would you correct or add?
Rx 3	Is this prescription ready to be processed and filled? Yes No What would you correct or add?
Rx 4	Is this prescription ready to be processed and filled? Yes No What would you correct or add?

Answer Key #2

Rx 1	Is this prescription ready to be processed and filled? No What would you correct or add? Wrong drug strength (10 mg) Add: Take at the same time every day
Rx 2	Is this prescription ready to be processed and filled? No What would you correct or add? Missing date Wrong drug form (Sporanox 100mg) Add: Take with a full meal
Rx 3	Is this prescription ready to be processed and filled? No What would you correct or add? Incomplete patient information (missing address) Wrong dosage (35mg/week) Add: Take on empty stomach with a full glass of water. Do not crush tablet. Do not lye down. Maintain upright position and empty stomach for at least 30 min.
Rx 4	Is this prescription ready to be processed and filled? No What would you correct or add? Wrong drug. Risperdal is antipsychotic.

Non Interactive Case #3: New Prescriptions Check

Candidate instructions:

Identify any mistakes, omissions or concerns on each new prescription. Some prescriptions have more than one problem. Omission of practitioner ID is not to be considered a mistake.
Use your answer sheet to record your answers. You have a total of **4 prescriptions** in this station.

Station Reference: CPS – Compendium of Pharmaceuticals and Specialties

You have 7 minutes to complete this station

Written Rx 1

Rx 1
Patient Name: Jaden Timmy
Address: 22 Hill Avenue

Correct date

Mevacor 40 mg
i tab once a day for 3 months

X. Kassam
_____ Assume signature is correct
X. Kassam M.D.

Written Rx 2

```
Rx 2
Patient Name: Cynthia Smith
Address: 675 Hill Way

                                        Correct date


      Adderall XR 10 mg
      PO 10 mg qd x 8 weeks for ADHD



         Y. Lee
   _____   Assume signature is correct
         Y. Lee M.D.
```

Written Rx 3

```
Rx 3
Patient Name: Josie and Tim Pearson
Address: 3-500 Sunny Bay


                                        Correct date

Adalat 90 mg
 i tab bid x 90 days for hypertension



         K. Said
   _____   Assume signature is correct
         K. Said M.D.
```

Written Rx 4

```
Rx 4
Patient Name: Ryan Kim
Address: 3590 3rd Road

                                                Correct date

     Actos
     One tablet daily for 3 months for diabetes



     _____          Assume signature is correct
          P. Sean M.D.
```

Answer Sheet: New Prescriptions Check

Rx 1	Is this prescription ready to be processed and filled? Yes No What would you correct or add?
Rx 2	Is this prescription ready to be processed and filled? Yes No What would you correct or add?
Rx 3	Is this prescription ready to be processed and filled? Yes No What would you correct or add?
Rx 4	Is this prescription ready to be processed and filled? Yes No What would you correct or add?

Answer Key #3

Rx 1	Is this prescription ready to be processed and filled? Yes What would you correct or add? Add: Take within evening meal
Rx 2	Is this prescription ready to be processed and filled? Yes What would you correct or add? Add: Take in the morning
Rx 3	Is this prescription ready to be processed and filled? No What would you correct or add? Two patients on the prescription Wrong dosage (once daily for 90 mg sustained release tablets) Add: Do not crush tablet; swallow whole.
Rx 4	Is this prescription ready to be processed and filled? No What would you correct or add? Missing drug strength Missing physician signature Add: take at the same time each day

Non Interactive Case #4: New Prescriptions Check

Candidate instructions:

Identify any mistakes, omissions or concerns on each new prescription. Some prescriptions have more than one problem. Omission of practitioner ID is not to be considered a mistake.
Use your answer sheet to record your answers. You have a total of **5 prescriptions** in this station.

Station Reference: CPS – Compendium of Pharmaceuticals and Specialties

You have 7 minutes to complete this station

Written Rx 1

```
Rx 1
Patient Name: Miranda Douglas
Address: 511 Victoria Street

                                                    Correct date
     Strattera 40 mg
     40 mg qd x 60 days for ADHD



         L Junior
   _____    Assume signature is correct
         L. Junior M.D.
```

Written Rx 2

> Rx 2
> Patient Name: Bob Singh
> Address: 4001 Simon Fraser Road
>
> Correct date
>
> Aldactone
> PO ii tabs qd x 2 weeks for edema
>
> *M Hamed*
> _____ Assume signature is correct
> M. Hamed M.D.

Written Rx 3

> Rx 3
> Patient Name: Pauline Maison
> Address: 444B Crescent
>
> Correct date
>
> Invega 90 mg
> 90 mg tab daily for 1 month for Schizophrenia
>
> *H. Tremblay*
> _____ Assume signature is correct
> H. Tremblay M.D.

Written Rx 4

```
Rx 4
Patient Name: Fanny Rock
Address: 7775 Hill Place

                                          Correct date

       Accolate 20 mg
       20 mg twice daily for 8 weeks



         K. Sunny
    _____      Assume signature is correct
         K. Sunny M.D.
```

Written Rx 5

```
Rx 5
Patient Name: Thomas Summer
Address: 9999 Hill Street

                                          Correct date

       Levitra 10 mg
       PO i tab before sexual activity
       Mitte: 60 tablets



         B. Bernard
    _____      Assume signature is correct
         B. Bernard M.D.
```

Answer Sheet: New Prescriptions Check

Rx 1	Is this prescription ready to be processed and filled? Yes　　　　　　　No What would you correct or add?
Rx 2	Is this prescription ready to be processed and filled? Yes　　　　　　　No What would you correct or add?
Rx 3	Is this prescription ready to be processed and filled? Yes　　　　　　　No What would you correct or add?
Rx 4	Is this prescription ready to be processed and filled? Yes　　　　　　　No What would you correct or add?
Rx 5	Is this prescription ready to be processed and filled? Yes　　　　　　　No What would you correct or add?

Answer Key #4

Rx 1	Is this prescription ready to be processed and filled? Yes What would you correct or add? Add: Take in the morning
Rx 2	Is this prescription ready to be processed and filled? No What would you correct or add? Missing drug strength Add: Take with food
Rx 3	Is this prescription ready to be processed and filled? No What would you correct or add? Wrong drug strength (9 mg) Add: Take ideally in the morning
Rx 4	Is this prescription ready to be processed and filled? Yes What would you correct or add? Add; Take on empty stomach
Rx 5	Is this prescription ready to be processed and filled? Yes What would you correct or add? Add: Take at least 30 min before sexual activity

Non Interactive Case #5: New Prescriptions Check

Candidate instructions:

Identify any mistakes, omissions or concerns on each new prescription. Some prescriptions have more than one problem. Omission of practitioner ID is not to be considered a mistake.
Use your answer sheet to record your answers. You have a total of **5 prescriptions** in this station.

Station Reference: CPS – Compendium of Pharmaceuticals and Specialties

You have 7 minutes to complete this station

Written Rx 1

Rx 1
Patient Name: Hanna Ryan
Address: 88C Winter Street

                                                                   Correct date

Inderal LA 120 mg
One cap once a day for 4 weeks for hypertension

N. Wong
_____ Assume signature is correct
N. Wong M.D.

Written Rx 2

```
Rx 2
Patient Name: Yan Lewis
Address: 350 Hall Street

                                              Correct date


       Malarone 250 mg/100mg
       PO i tab qd for the prevention of malaria
       Starting 1 to 2 days before travel and continuing for 7 days after
       leaving the affected area.


         K. Mason
_____   Assume signature is correct
         K. Mason M.D.
```

Written Rx 3

```
Rx 3
Patient Name: April Park
Address: 35 Oak Bay

                                              Correct date


       Lipitor 40 mg
       One tablet for 3 months for hypercholesterolemia



         G. Ali
_____   Assume signature is correct
         G. Ali M.D.
```

Written Rx 4

```
Rx 4
Patient Name: David Olsen
Address: 442 2nd Street

                                              Correct date

     Femara 2.5 mg
     PO i tab once a day for breast cancer
     Mitte: 90 days


         O.Albanny
    _____   Assume signature is correct
         O. Albanny M.D.
```

Written Rx 5

```
Rx 5
Patient Name: Miranda Josef
Address: 35 Canada Way

                                              Correct date

Avelox 5%
1 drop in both ears tid for 7 days



         W. George
    _____   Assume signature is correct
         W. George M.D.
```

Answer Sheet: New Prescriptions Check

Rx 1	Is this prescription ready to be processed and filled? Yes No What would you correct or add?
Rx 2	Is this prescription ready to be processed and filled? Yes No What would you correct or add?
Rx 3	Is this prescription ready to be processed and filled? Yes No What would you correct or add?
Rx 4	Is this prescription ready to be processed and filled? Yes No What would you correct or add?
Rx 5	Is this prescription ready to be processed and filled? Yes No What would you correct or add?

Answer Key #5

Rx 1	Is this prescription ready to be processed and filled? Yes What would you correct or add? Add: Take at bedtime
Rx 2	Is this prescription ready to be processed and filled? Yes What would you correct or add? Add: Take with food.
Rx 3	Is this prescription ready to be processed and filled? Yes What would you correct or add?
Rx 4	Is this prescription ready to be processed and filled? Yes What would you correct or add? Add: Take at the same time each day
Rx 5	Is this prescription ready to be processed and filled? No What would you correct or add? Wrong drug strength (0.5% solution) Wrong administration route (eyes)

Non Interactive Case #6: New Prescriptions Check

Candidate instructions:

Identify any mistakes, omissions or concerns on each new prescription. Some prescriptions have more than one problem. Omission of practitioner ID is not to be considered a mistake.
Use your answer sheet to record your answers. You have a total of **3 prescriptions** in this station.

Station Reference: CPS – Compendium of Pharmaceuticals and Specialties

You have 7 minutes to complete this station

Written Rx 1

Rx 1
Patient Name: Veronica Sam
Address: 234th Street

                                                        Correct date

   Xenical
   120 mg cap i tid for 12 months

   T. June
   _____   Assume signature is correct
   T. June M.D.

Written Rx 2

```
Rx 2
Patient Name: Tannis Moon
Address: 34A Street

                                              Correct date


        Meridia
        10 mg once a day
        Mitte: 30 tablets


          N. Smith
    _____    Assume signature is correct
        N. Smith M.D.
```

Written Rx 3

```
Rx 3
Patient Name: Min Kim
Address: Heron Road




        Betaloc
        50 mg qid x 6 months



          P. Wong
    _____    Assume signature is correct
        P. Wong M.D.
```

Answer Sheet: New Prescriptions Check

Rx 1	Is this prescription ready to be processed and filled? Yes No What would you correct or add?
Rx 2	Is this prescription ready to be processed and filled? Yes No What would you correct or add?
Rx 3	Is this prescription ready to be processed and filled? Yes No What would you correct or add?

Answer Key #6

Rx 1	Is this prescription ready to be processed and filled? Yes What would you correct or add? Add: Take with or up to 1 hour after a meal containing fat.
Rx 2	Is this prescription ready to be processed and filled? Yes What would you correct or add?
Rx 3	Is this prescription ready to be processed and filled? No What would you correct or add? Missing date

Non Interactive Case #7: New Prescriptions Check

Candidate instructions:

Identify any mistakes, omissions or concerns on each new prescription. Some prescriptions have more than one problem. Omission of practitioner ID is not to be considered a mistake.
Use your answer sheet to record your answers. You have a total of **3 prescriptions** in this station.

Station Reference: CPS – Compendium of Pharmaceuticals and Specialties

You have 7 minutes to complete this station

Written Rx 1

```
Rx 1
Patient Name: Ann John
Address: 223B Street

                                              Correct date


        Actos
        30 mg tid x 6 weeks




        N. John
   _____    Assume signature is correct
        N. John M.D.
```

Written Rx 2

```
Rx 2
Patient Name: Karen Simon
Address:
                                           Correct date


       Glucophage
       1500 mg daily divided tid x 6 months




         P. Ahmed
    _____  Assume signature is correct
         P. Ahmed M.D.
```

Written Rx 3

```
Rx 3
Patient Name: Paul Ryan
Address: 8 Royal Avenue
                                           Correct date


       Diamicron MR
       120 mg twice a day
       Mitte: 60 tablets




         N. Wen
    _____  Assume signature is correct
         N. Wen M.D.
```

Answer Sheet: New Prescriptions Check

Rx 1	Is this prescription ready to be processed and filled? Yes No What would you correct or add?
Rx 2	Is this prescription ready to be processed and filled? Yes No What would you correct or add?
Rx 3	Is this prescription ready to be processed and filled? Yes No What would you correct or add?

Answer Key #7

Rx 1	Is this prescription ready to be processed and filled? No What would you correct or add? Wrong dosage. It is once daily.
Rx 2	Is this prescription ready to be processed and filled? No What would you correct or add? Missing address
Rx 3	Is this prescription ready to be processed and filled? No What would you correct or add? Wrong dosage. Once a day for long acting gliclazide

Non Interactive Case #8: New Prescriptions Check

Candidate instructions:

Identify any mistakes, omissions or concerns on each new prescription. Some prescriptions have more than one problem. Omission of practitioner ID is not to be considered a mistake.
Use your answer sheet to record your answers. You have a total of **3 prescriptions** in this station.

Station Reference: CPS – Compendium of Pharmaceuticals and Specialties

You have 7 minutes to complete this station

Written Rx 1

Rx 1
Patient Name: Kim Spring
Address: 12 Skye Avenue

Correct date

GlucoNorm
2 mg once a day x 4 months

N. Ali
_____ Assume signature is correct
N. Ali M.D.

Written Rx 2

```
Rx 2
Patient Name: Mary Park
Address: 341 Montreal Street

                                          Correct date


          Crestor
          20 mg once a day for 1 year



            G. Norm
    _____    Assume signature is correct
           G. Norm M.D.
```

Written Rx 3

```
Rx 3
Patient Name: Amanda Thomas
Address: 215D Street

                                          Correct date


          Lipidil Supra
          160 mg daily for hyperlipidemia for 2 months



            N. Kim
    _____    Assume signature is correct
           N. Kim M.D.
```

Answer Sheet: New Prescriptions Check

Rx 1	Is this prescription ready to be processed and filled? Yes No What would you correct or add?
Rx 2	Is this prescription ready to be processed and filled? Yes No What would you correct or add?
Rx 3	Is this prescription ready to be processed and filled? Yes No What would you correct or add?

Answer Key #8

Rx 1	Is this prescription ready to be processed and filled? Yes What would you correct or add? Add: Take within 30 min of beginning of a meal
Rx 2	Is this prescription ready to be processed and filled? Yes What would you correct or add? Add: Do not take within 2 hours of taking an antacid
Rx 3	Is this prescription ready to be processed and filled? Yes What would you correct or add? Add: Take with largest meal of the day

Non Interactive Case #9: New Prescriptions Check

Candidate instructions:

Identify any mistakes, omissions or concerns on each new prescription. Some prescriptions have more than one problem. Omission of practitioner ID is not to be considered a mistake.
Use your answer sheet to record your answers. You have a total of **3 prescriptions** in this station.

Station Reference: CPS – Compendium of Pharmaceuticals and Specialties

You have 7 minutes to complete this station

Written Rx 1

Rx 1
Patient Name: Vera Gill
Address: 21 King Street

Correct date

Tylenol #3
1 tablet every 6 hours is needed for pain
Mitte: 30 tablets

_____   Assume signature is correct
N. Jim M.D.

Written Rx 2

> Rx 2
> Patient Name: Patrick Neil
> Address: 34 2nd Avenue
>
>   Correct date
>
>   Imdur
>   Once a day for angina
>   Mitte: 8 weeks
>
>   *W. Vohn*
> _____ Assume signature is correct
>   W. Vohn M.D.

Written Rx 3

> Rx 3
> Patient Name: Meena Singh
> Address: 45 Union Square
>
>   Correct date
>
>   Nitrol
>   1 spray Q5min prn for angina pain x 2 months
>
>   *D. Moon*
> _____ Assume signature is correct
>   D. Moon M.D.

Answer Sheet: New Prescriptions Check

Rx 1	Is this prescription ready to be processed and filled? Yes　　　　　　　No What would you correct or add?
Rx 2	Is this prescription ready to be processed and filled? Yes　　　　　　　No What would you correct or add?
Rx 3	Is this prescription ready to be processed and filled? Yes　　　　　　　No What would you correct or add?

Answer Key #9

Rx 1	Is this prescription ready to be processed and filled? No What would you correct or add? Missing physician signature
Rx 2	Is this prescription ready to be processed and filled? No What would you correct or add? Missing dosage.
Rx 3	Is this prescription ready to be processed and filled? No What would you correct or add? Wrong drug. Nitrol is nitroglycerin ointment not a spray.

Non Interactive Case #10: New Prescriptions Check

Candidate instructions:

Identify any mistakes, omissions or concerns on each new prescription. Some prescriptions have more than one problem. Omission of practitioner ID is not to be considered a mistake.
Use your answer sheet to record your answers. You have a total of **3 prescriptions** in this station.

Station Reference: CPS – Compendium of Pharmaceuticals and Specialties

You have 7 minutes to complete this station

Written Rx 1

Rx 1
Patient Name: Susan Kim
Address: 43B Street

                                                        Correct date

     Kineret
     100 mg po daily for rheumatoid arthritis
     Mitte: 4 weeks

     R. Khalid
_____   Assume signature is correct
     R. Khalid M.D.

Written Rx 2

```
Rx 2
Patient Name: Catherine Jones
Address: 2112 One Street

                                        Correct date


     Miacalcin NS
     200 IU daily intranasal x 1 month



        H. Loo
_____     Assume signature is correct
     H. Loo M.D.
```

Written Rx 3

```
Rx 3
Patient Name: Liam and Jane Simmis
Address: Laval Street

                                        Correct date


     Zovirax
     400 mg tid for genital herpes
     Mitte: 1 week



        R. Kassam
_____     Assume signature is correct
     R. Kassam M.D.
```

Answer Sheet: New Prescriptions Check

Rx 1	Is this prescription ready to be processed and filled? Yes No What would you correct or add?
Rx 2	Is this prescription ready to be processed and filled? Yes No What would you correct or add?
Rx 3	Is this prescription ready to be processed and filled? Yes No What would you correct or add?

Answer Key #10

Rx 1	Is this prescription ready to be processed and filled? No What would you correct or add? Wrong administration route. Anakinra (Kineret) is administrated by sc.
Rx 2	Is this prescription ready to be processed and filled? Yes What would you correct or add? Add : Prime before first use. Spray in one nostril.
Rx 3	Is this prescription ready to be processed and filled? No What would you correct or add? Two patients on the same prescription.

Non Interactive Case #11: New Prescriptions Check

Candidate instructions:

Identify any mistakes, omissions or concerns on each new prescription. Some prescriptions have more than one problem. Omission of practitioner ID is not to be considered a mistake.
Use your answer sheet to record your answers. You have a total of **3 prescriptions** in this station.

Station Reference: CPS – Compendium of Pharmaceuticals and Specialties

You have 7 minutes to complete this station

Written Rx 1

Rx 1
Patient Name: Karyn Peter
Address: Ottawa Street

Prozac
20 mg once a day
Mitte: 8 weeks

N. Simon
_____ Assume signature is correct
N. Simon M.D.

Written Rx 2

```
Rx 2
Patient Name: Dan Summer
Address:  Morning Street

                                            Correct date


     5-Fluorouracil cream
      Apply twice a day for 4 weeks



        L. James
                                      Assume signature is correct
  _____
        L. James M.D.
```

Written Rx 3

```
Rx 3
Patient Name: Joe Ryan
Address:  Kamloops Avenue

                                            Correct date


     Timoptic-XE
     0.5% solution 1 drop in left eye twice a day for 8 weeks



        T. Farid
                                      Assume signature is correct
  _____
        T. Farid M.D.
```

Answer Sheet: New Prescriptions Check

Rx 1	Is this prescription ready to be processed and filled? Yes No What would you correct or add?
Rx 2	Is this prescription ready to be processed and filled? Yes No What would you correct or add?
Rx 3	Is this prescription ready to be processed and filled? Yes No What would you correct or add?

Answer Key #11

Rx 1	Is this prescription ready to be processed and filled? No What would you correct or add? Missing date Add: Take in the morning.
Rx 2	Is this prescription ready to be processed and filled? No What would you correct or add? Missing strength. Add: Apply with gloved fingers.
Rx 3	Is this prescription ready to be processed and filled? No What would you correct or add? Wrong dosage. Once a day dosing for Timoptic-XE

Non Interactive Case #12: New Prescriptions Check

Candidate instructions:

Identify any mistakes, omissions or concerns on each new prescription. Some prescriptions have more than one problem. Omission of practitioner ID is not to be considered a mistake.
Use your answer sheet to record your answers. You have a total of **3 prescriptions** in this station.

Station Reference: CPS – Compendium of Pharmaceuticals and Specialties

You have 7 minutes to complete this station

Written Rx 1

Rx 1
Patient Name: Karim Hassan
Address: 34 Canada Blvd

Correct date

Abilify
15 mg once a day
Mitte: 4 weeks

J. Peter
_____ Assume signature is correct
J. Peter M.D.

Written Rx 2

```
Rx 2
Patient Name: Wayne Folgers
Address: 211 Avenue

                                          Correct date


       Accolate
       20 mg BID for asthma
       Mitte: 30 days


          N. Lam
       _____      Assume signature is correct
         N. Lam M.D.
```

Written Rx 3

```
Rx 3
Patient Name: Von Smith
Address: 21A Street

                                          Correct date


       Accuretic
       20/25 tab i qid x 3 months


          N. Jim
       _____      Assume signature is correct
         N. Jim M.D.
```

Answer Sheet: New Prescriptions Check

Rx 1	Is this prescription ready to be processed and filled? Yes　　　　　　No What would you correct or add?
Rx 2	Is this prescription ready to be processed and filled? Yes　　　　　　No What would you correct or add?
Rx 3	Is this prescription ready to be processed and filled? Yes　　　　　　No What would you correct or add?

Answer Key #12

Rx 1	Is this prescription ready to be processed and filled? Yes What would you correct or add?
Rx 2	Is this prescription ready to be processed and filled? Yes What would you correct or add? Add: Take one hour before or 2 hours after meals
Rx 3	Is this prescription ready to be processed and filled? No What would you correct or add? Wrong dosage

Non Interactive Case #13: New Prescriptions Check

Candidate instructions:

Identify any mistakes, omissions or concerns on each new prescription. Some prescriptions have more than one problem. Omission of practitioner ID is not to be considered a mistake.
Use your answer sheet to record your answers. You have a total of **3 prescriptions** in this station.

Station Reference: CPS – Compendium of Pharmaceuticals and Specialties

You have 7 minutes to complete this station

Written Rx 1

Rx 1
Patient Name: Keelan Kim
Address: 6 Sunny Avenue

Correct date

Actonel DR
1 tablet in the morning with breakfast once a week
Mitte: 24 tablets

P. Singh
_____ Assume signature is correct
P. Singh M.D.

Written Rx 2

```
Rx 2
Patient Name: Ben Hamed
Address: 12 Vancouver Street

                                        Correct date


    Adalat XL
    30 mg once a day
    Mitte: 6 months


         A.   Hammond
    _____    Assume signature is correct
       A. Hammond M.D.
```

Written Rx 3

```
Rx 3
Patient Name: Patience Pena
Address: 9 Calgary Drive

                                        Correct date


    Aggrenox
    200/25 cap i bid
    Mitte: 60 tablets


         N. Wayne
    _____    Assume signature is correct
       N. Wayne M.D.
```

Answer Sheet: New Prescriptions Check

Rx 1	Is this prescription ready to be processed and filled? Yes No What would you correct or add?
Rx 2	Is this prescription ready to be processed and filled? Yes No What would you correct or add?
Rx 3	Is this prescription ready to be processed and filled? Yes No What would you correct or add?

Answer Key #13

Rx 1	Is this prescription ready to be processed and filled? Yes What would you correct or add? Add: Swallow the tablet whole with plenty of water; do not chew, crush or cut. Do not lie down for at least 30 min.
Rx 2	Is this prescription ready to be processed and filled? Yes What would you correct or add? Add: Swallow the tablet whole.
Rx 3	Is this prescription ready to be processed and filled? Yes What would you correct or add? Add: Swallow the tablet whole, do not chew.

Non Interactive Case #14: New Prescriptions Check

Candidate instructions:

Identify any mistakes, omissions or concerns on each new prescription. Some prescriptions have more than one problem. Omission of practitioner ID is not to be considered a mistake.
Use your answer sheet to record your answers. You have a total of **3 prescriptions** in this station.

Station Reference: CPS – Compendium of Pharmaceuticals and Specialties

You have 7 minutes to complete this station

Written Rx 1

Rx 1
Patient Name: Bob Murphy
Address: 56 3rd Avenue

Correct date

Ampicillin
250 mg q6h x 7 days

J. Young
_____ Assume signature is correct
J. Young M.D.

Written Rx 2

```
Rx 2
Patient Name:
Address: 3 Hope Street

                                          Correct date


     Betagan 0.5%
     1 spray in each nostril twice a day for 7 days


        N. John
     _____    Assume signature is correct
        N. John M.D.
```

Written Rx 3

```
Rx 3
Patient Name: Don Reid
Address: 2 Winter Avenue

                                          Correct date


     Cardizem
     30 mg for angina
     Mitte: 3 months


        R. Lee
     _____    Assume signature is correct
        R. Lee M.D.
```

Answer Sheet: New Prescriptions Check

Rx 1	Is this prescription ready to be processed and filled? Yes No What would you correct or add?
Rx 2	Is this prescription ready to be processed and filled? Yes No What would you correct or add?
Rx 3	Is this prescription ready to be processed and filled? Yes No What would you correct or add?

Answer Key #14

Rx 1	Is this prescription ready to be processed and filled? Yes What would you correct or add? Add: Take on empty stomach, one hour before or two hours after a meal
Rx 2	Is this prescription ready to be processed and filled? No What would you correct or add? Missing patient's name and wrong route of administration. Betagan is an ophthalmic solution.
Rx 3	Is this prescription ready to be processed and filled? No What would you correct or add? Incomplete dosing information.

Non Interactive Case #15: New Prescriptions Check

Candidate instructions:

Identify any mistakes, omissions or concerns on each new prescription. Some prescriptions have more than one problem. Omission of practitioner ID is not to be considered a mistake.
Use your answer sheet to record your answers. You have a total of **3 prescriptions** in this station.

Station Reference: CPS – Compendium of Pharmaceuticals and Specialties

You have 7 minutes to complete this station

Written Rx 1

```
Rx 1
Patient Name: Richard Tim
Address: 7 Noon Drive

                                        Correct date


        Paxil CR
        25 mg daily in the morning for 30 days for depression




        _____          Assume signature is correct
        N. Gold M.D.
```

Written Rx 2

```
Rx 2
Patient Name: Summer Joe
Address: 21 Spring Way

                                          Correct date


       Ceftin suspension
       125 mg q12h for 5 days


           Y. Long
       _____   Assume signature is correct
           Y. Long M.D.
```

Written Rx 3

```
Rx 3
Patient Name: Sharon Dylan
Address: 21 Funny Drive

                                          Correct date


       Buspirone
       10 mg tablet twice a day for 3 weeks


           N. Habib
       _____   Assume signature is correct
           N. Habib M.D.
```

Answer Sheet: New Prescriptions Check

Rx 1	Is this prescription ready to be processed and filled? Yes　　　　　　　　No What would you correct or add?
Rx 2	Is this prescription ready to be processed and filled? Yes　　　　　　　　No What would you correct or add?
Rx 3	Is this prescription ready to be processed and filled? Yes　　　　　　　　No What would you correct or add?

Answer Key #15

Rx 1	Is this prescription ready to be processed and filled? No What would you correct or add? Missing physician signature. Add: Swallow the tablet whole, do not crush or chew.
Rx 2	Is this prescription ready to be processed and filled? Yes What would you correct or add? Add: Shake well before use.
Rx 3	Is this prescription ready to be processed and filled? Yes What would you correct or add? Add: Avoid grapefruit juice.

Non Interactive Case #16: New Prescriptions Check

Candidate instructions:

Identify any mistakes, omissions or concerns on each new prescription. Some prescriptions have more than one problem. Omission of practitioner ID is not to be considered a mistake.
Use your answer sheet to record your answers. You have a total of **3 prescriptions** in this station.

Station Reference: CPS – Compendium of Pharmaceuticals and Specialties

You have 7 minutes to complete this station

Written Rx 1

Rx 1
Patient Name: Gurpreet Gill
Address: 3 Summer Road

Correct date

Bezalip SR
400 mg once a day
Mitte: 60 tablets

T. Thomas
_____ Assume signature is correct
T. Thomas M.D.

Written Rx 2

```
Rx 2
Patient Name: Rick John
Address: 21B Avenue

                                           Correct date


    Cipro
    500 mg for 8 days


       N. Smith
    _____   Assume signature is correct
       N. Smith M.D.
```

Written Rx 3

```
Rx 3
Patient Name: June Park
Address: One Drive

                                           Correct date


    Xalacom
    Apply ½ inch ointment to affected area twice a day for 7 days
    Mitte: 30g


       P. Dean
    _____   Assume signature is correct
       P. Dean M.D.
```

Answer Sheet: New Prescriptions Check

Rx 1	Is this prescription ready to be processed and filled? Yes No What would you correct or add?
Rx 2	Is this prescription ready to be processed and filled? Yes No What would you correct or add?
Rx 3	Is this prescription ready to be processed and filled? Yes No What would you correct or add?

Answer Key #16

Rx 1	Is this prescription ready to be processed and filled? Yes What would you correct or add? Add: Take in the morning or evening with or after meals. Swallow the tablet whole with sufficient liquid.
Rx 2	Is this prescription ready to be processed and filled? No What would you correct or add? Incomplete dosing information. Add: Take at least 2 hours before or 6 hours after an antacid and supplements containing ions such as magnesium, aluminum, iron and zinc.
Rx 3	Is this prescription ready to be processed and filled? No What would you correct or add? Wrong drug. Xalacom is an ophthalmic drug.

Non Interactive Case #17: New Prescriptions Check

Candidate instructions:

Identify any mistakes, omissions or concerns on each new prescription. Some prescriptions have more than one problem. Omission of practitioner ID is not to be considered a mistake.
Use your answer sheet to record your answers. You have a total of **3 prescriptions** in this station.

Station Reference: CPS – Compendium of Pharmaceuticals and Specialties

You have 7 minutes to complete this station

Written Rx 1

Rx 1
Patient Name: Mary and Ryan Paul
Address:

Correct date

Sporanox
100 mg cap daily for oral candidiasis
Mitte: 2 weeks

T. Thomas
_____   Assume signature is correct
T. Thomas M.D.

Written Rx 2

```
Rx 2
Patient Name: Cynthia James
Address: 5 Snow Street

                                    Correct date


        Clomiphene
        50 mg cap twice a day for OCD
        Mitte: 4 weeks



           L. Goa
        _____    Assume signature is correct
           L. Goa M.D.
```

Written Rx 3

```
Rx 3
Patient Name: Kate Sperling
Address: Primary Avenue

                                    Correct date


        Pilocarpine
        1 drop in both eyes three times a day for 7 days


           Y. Min
        _____    Assume signature is correct
           Y. Min M.D.
```

Answer Sheet: New Prescriptions Check

Rx 1	Is this prescription ready to be processed and filled? Yes No What would you correct or add?
Rx 2	Is this prescription ready to be processed and filled? Yes No What would you correct or add?
Rx 3	Is this prescription ready to be processed and filled? Yes No What would you correct or add?

Answer Key #17

Rx 1	Is this prescription ready to be processed and filled? No What would you correct or add? Incomplete patient's information, missing address. More than one person per prescription.
Rx 2	Is this prescription ready to be processed and filled? No What would you correct or add? Wrong drug. Clomiphene and chlomipramine are sound-alike medications.
Rx 3	Is this prescription ready to be processed and filled? No What would you correct or add? Missing drug strength.

Non Interactive Case #18: New Prescriptions Check

Candidate instructions:

Identify any mistakes, omissions or concerns on each new prescription. Some prescriptions have more than one problem. Omission of practitioner ID is not to be considered a mistake.
Use your answer sheet to record your answers. You have a total of **3 prescriptions** in this station.

Station Reference: CPS – Compendium of Pharmaceuticals and Specialties

You have 7 minutes to complete this station

Written Rx 1

Rx 1
Patient Name: James Peter
Address: 89 Laval Street

Correct date

Sinequan
50 mg once a day
Mitte: 30 tablets

N. Dylan
_____   Assume signature is correct
N. Dylan M.D.

Written Rx 2

```
Rx 2
Patient Name: Jane Bryan
Address: 55D Square

                                          Correct date


      Buspirone
      150 mg once a day for 3 days for smoking cessation


         G. Bolt
      _____  Assume signature is correct
         G. Bolt M.D.
```

Written Rx 3

```
Rx 3
Patient Name: Veera Johns
Address: 676 Quebec Street

                                          Correct date


      Lyrica
      150 mg bid for neuropathic pain
      Mitte: 8 weeks


         R. Smith
      _____  Assume signature is correct
         R. Smith M.D.
```

Answer Sheet: New Prescriptions Check

Rx 1	Is this prescription ready to be processed and filled? Yes No What would you correct or add?
Rx 2	Is this prescription ready to be processed and filled? Yes No What would you correct or add?
Rx 3	Is this prescription ready to be processed and filled? Yes No What would you correct or add?

Answer Key #18

Rx 1	Is this prescription ready to be processed and filled? Yes What would you correct or add? Add: Take at bedtime. Avoid alcohol.
Rx 2	Is this prescription ready to be processed and filled? No What would you correct or add? Wrong drug. Bupropion and buspirone are sound-alike drugs
Rx 3	Is this prescription ready to be processed and filled? Yes What would you correct or add?

Non Interactive Case #19: New Prescriptions Check

Candidate instructions:

Identify any mistakes, omissions or concerns on each new prescription. Some prescriptions have more than one problem. Omission of practitioner ID is not to be considered a mistake.
Use your answer sheet to record your answers. You have a total of **3 prescriptions** in this station.

Station Reference: CPS – Compendium of Pharmaceuticals and Specialties

You have 7 minutes to complete this station

Written Rx 1

```
Rx 1
Patient Name: Cathy Fong
Address: 21 2nd street

                                              Correct date


       Cortenema
       100 mg po once a day at bedtime for IBS
       Mitte: 4 weeks



         H. Kong
       _____    Assume signature is correct
         H. Kong M.D.
```

Written Rx 2

```
Rx 2
Patient Name: Mimi Kim
Address: 55 Angela Street

                                        Correct date


     Zocor
     40 mg once a day for hyperlidemia
     Mitte: 3 months


        O. Salem
     _____    Assume signature is correct
        O. Salem M.D.
```

Written Rx 3

```
Rx 3
Patient Name: Norman Simms
Address: 213 3rd avenue

                                        Correct date


     Topamax
     400 mg for seizures
     Mitte: 12 weeks


        D. Paul
     _____    Assume signature is correct
        D. Paul M.D.
```

Answer Sheet: New Prescriptions Check

Rx 1	Is this prescription ready to be processed and filled? Yes No What would you correct or add?
Rx 2	Is this prescription ready to be processed and filled? Yes No What would you correct or add?
Rx 3	Is this prescription ready to be processed and filled? Yes No What would you corrcct or add?

Answer Key #19

Rx 1	Is this prescription ready to be processed and filled? No What would you correct or add? Wrong administration route. Cortenema is administered as enema.
Rx 2	Is this prescription ready to be processed and filled? Yes What would you correct or add? Add: Take with evening meal.
Rx 3	Is this prescription ready to be processed and filled? No What would you correct or add? Missing dosing information. Add: Do not chew tablets because of bitter taste.

Non Interactive Case #20: New Prescriptions Check

Candidate instructions:

Identify any mistakes, omissions or concerns on each new prescription. Some prescriptions have more than one problem. Omission of practitioner ID is not to be considered a mistake.
Use your answer sheet to record your answers. You have a total of **3 prescriptions** in this station.

Station Reference: CPS – Compendium of Pharmaceuticals and Specialties

You have 7 minutes to complete this station

Written Rx 1

Rx 1
Patient Name: Karyn Smith
Address: Toronto Street

                                                                                   Correct date

        Imitrex
        100 mg may repeat in 30 min for migraine headache pain
        Mitte: 60 tablets

        N. Cairn
_____ Assume signature is correct
    N. Cairn M.D.

Written Rx 2

```
Rx 2
Patient Name: Thomas Young
Address: 21B Avenue

                                          Correct date


     Cardura
     1 tablet once a day for hypertension
     Mitte: 30 tablets


         G. Wang
     _____    Assume signature is correct
         G. Wang M.D.
```

Written Rx 3

```
Rx 3
Patient Name: Fanny and Joe Pete
Address: 2123 Street

                                          Correct date


     Sibelium
     5 mg once a day x 4 weeks for headache


         F. Tom
     _____    Assume signature is correct
         F. Tom M.D.
```

Answer Sheet: New Prescriptions Check

Rx 1	Is this prescription ready to be processed and filled? Yes No What would you correct or add?
Rx 2	Is this prescription ready to be processed and filled? Yes No What would you correct or add?
Rx 3	Is this prescription ready to be processed and filled? Yes No What would you correct or add?

Answer Key #20

Rx 1	Is this prescription ready to be processed and filled? No What would you correct or add? Wrong dosing. May repeat in 2 hours. Add: Do not exceed 200 mg a day.
Rx 2	Is this prescription ready to be processed and filled? No What would you correct or add? Missing tablet strength. Add: Take initial dose at bedtime to prevent syncope.
Rx 3	Is this prescription ready to be processed and filled? No What would you correct or add? More than one person per order

Non Interactive Case #21: New Prescriptions Check

Candidate instructions:

Identify any mistakes, omissions or concerns on each new prescription. Some prescriptions have more than one problem. Omission of practitioner ID is not to be considered a mistake.
Use your answer sheet to record your answers. You have a total of **4 prescriptions** in this station.

Station Reference: CPS – Compendium of Pharmaceuticals and Specialties

You have 7 minutes to complete this station

Written Rx 1

> Rx 1
> Patient Name: Simon Brett
> Address: 23th Street
>
> Correct date
>
> Cholestyramine
> 4g bid x 4 months
>
> _____   Assume signature is correct
> T. Jeremy M.D.

Written Rx 2

```
Rx 2
Patient Name: Pat Gill
Address: 34A Road

                                              Correct date


        Transderm V
        1 patch q24x 6 days



           N. Peter
_____  Assume signature is correct
         N. Peter
```

Written Rx 3

```
Rx 3
Patient Name: Miranda Kim
Address: Bear Road

                                              Correct date


        Ezetrol
        10 mg once daily at anytime for 12 weeks
        Mitte: 86 tablets


           P. Hamed
_____  Assume signature is correct
         P. Hamed M.D.
```

Written Rx 4

Rx 4
Patient Name: Rosie Kyhan
Address: 23 Summit Street

Correct date

Oxytrol 36 mg oxybutynin patch
Apply 1 patch each week for 12 weeks for incontinence

I. Chris
_____ Assume signature is correct
I. Chris M.D.

Answer Sheet: New Prescriptions Check

Rx 1	Is this prescription ready to be processed and filled? Yes No What would you correct or add?
Rx 2	Is this prescription ready to be processed and filled? Yes No What would you correct or add?
Rx 3	Is this prescription ready to be processed and filled? Yes No What would you correct or add?
Rx 4	Is this prescription ready to be processed and filled? Yes No What would you correct or add?

Answer Key #21

Rx 1	Is this prescription ready to be processed and filled? No What would you correct or add? Missing physician's signature Add: 1 hour or 4-6 hours after other medications. Increase fiber and fluid intake to prevent constipation.
Rx 2	Is this prescription ready to be processed and filled? No What would you correct or add? Wrong dosing. 1 patch q72h. 1.5 mg patch. Add: apply the patch behind the ear.
Rx 3	Is this prescription ready to be processed and filled? No What would you correct or add? Wrong number of tablets
Rx 4	Is this prescription ready to be processed and filled? No What would you correct or add? Wrong dosing. The patch is applied twice weekly.

Non Interactive Case #22: New Prescriptions Check

Candidate instructions:

Identify any mistakes, omissions or concerns on each new prescription. Some prescriptions have more than one problem. Omission of practitioner ID is not to be considered a mistake.
Use your answer sheet to record your answers. You have a total of **4 prescriptions** in this station.

Station Reference: CPS – Compendium of Pharmaceuticals and Specialties

You have 7 minutes to complete this station

Written Rx 1

Rx 1
Patient Name: Diane John
Address: Calgary Avenue

Correct date

Lopid
600 mg cap bid for 5 months
Mitte: 300 capsules

R. June
_____   Assume signature is correct
R. June M.D.

Written Rx 2

```
Rx 2
Patient Name: April Young
Address: Vancouver Avenue

                                          Correct date


       Livostin 0.5 mg/ml
       2 spays in each nostril bid


         O. Park
       _____   Assume signature is correct
         O. Park M.D.
```

Written Rx 3

```
Rx 3
Patient Name: Mary Koo
Address: High Road

                                          Correct date


       Cardizem CD
       180 mg for Raynaud's Syndrome



         P. Yan
       _____   Assume signature is correct
         P. Yan M.D.
```

Written Rx 4

Rx 4
Patient Name: Tannis Moon
Address: 34A Street

Correct date

Cimetidine
800 mg hs x 3 months for duodenal ulcer

N. Smith
_____ Assume signature is correct
N. Smith M.D.

Answer Sheet: New Prescriptions Check

Rx 1	Is this prescription ready to be processed and filled? Yes No What would you correct or add?
Rx 2	Is this prescription ready to be processed and filled? Yes No What would you correct or add?
Rx 3	Is this prescription ready to be processed and filled? Yes No What would you correct or add?
Rx 4	Is this prescription ready to be processed and filled? Yes No What would you correct or add?

Answer Key #22

Rx 1	Is this prescription ready to be processed and filled? Yes What would you correct or add? Add: Take 30 minutes prior to meals
Rx 2	Is this prescription ready to be processed and filled? Yes Add: Shake well before use. Prime before first use. Discontinue is no improvement after 3 days of use.
Rx 3	Is this prescription ready to be processed and filled? Yes What would you correct or add? Add: 60 to 90 minutes before exposure to cold.
Rx 4	Is this prescription ready to be processed and filled? Yes What would you correct or add? Add: Take 1 hour before or 2 hours after an antacid.

Non Interactive Case #23: New Prescriptions Check

Candidate instructions:

Identify any mistakes, omissions or concerns on each new prescription. Some prescriptions have more than one problem. Omission of practitioner ID is not to be considered a mistake.
Use your answer sheet to record your answers. You have a total of **4 prescriptions** in this station.

Station Reference: CPS – Compendium of Pharmaceuticals and Specialties

You have 7 minutes to complete this station

Written Rx 1

```
Rx 1
Patient Name: Samantha Roger
Address: 4th Street

                                          Correct date


        Mometasone 1%
        Apply to affected skin area once daily for 1 week
        Mitte: 15 g



        K. Lee
        _____      Assume signature is correct
        K. Lee M.D.
```

Written Rx 2

```
Rx 2
Patient Name: Tia Morning
Address: 34A Street

                                    Correct date


    Diovan
    160 mg once daily for 90 days
    Mitte: 90 tablets


       N. Smith
    _____    Assume signature is correct
       N. Smith M.D.
```

Written Rx 3

```
Rx 3
Patient Name: Karyn Parson
Address: 11 Summer Road

                                    Correct date


    Altace 5/25
    1 tab once daily x 12 weeks


       P. Mills
    _____    Assume signature is correct
       P. Mills M.D.
```

Written Rx 4

Rx 4
Patient Name: David Fong
Address: 87 Commercial Road

Correct date

Cialis
10 mg tab po 20 min before sexual activity
Mitte: 50 tablets

P. Wong
_____   Assume signature is correct
P. Wong M.D.

Answer Sheet: New Prescriptions Check

Rx 1	Is this prescription ready to be processed and filled? Yes No What would you correct or add?
Rx 2	Is this prescription ready to be processed and filled? Yes No What would you correct or add?
Rx 3	Is this prescription ready to be processed and filled? Yes No What would you correct or add?
Rx 4	Is this prescription ready to be processed and filled? Yes No What would you correct or add?

Answer Key #23

Rx 1	Is this prescription ready to be processed and filled? No What would you correct or add? Wrong drug strength.
Rx 2	Is this prescription ready to be processed and filled? Yes What would you correct or add? Take consistently with or without food.
Rx 3	Is this prescription ready to be processed and filled? Yes What would you correct or add? Add: Take in the morning. Swallow whole.
Rx 4	Is this prescription ready to be processed and filled? No What would you correct or add? Wrong dosing. Cialis is taken at least 60 minutes before sexual activity. Do not take more than every 2nd day.

Non Interactive Case #24: New Prescriptions Check

Candidate instructions:

Identify any mistakes, omissions or concerns on each new prescription. Some prescriptions have more than one problem. Omission of practitioner ID is not to be considered a mistake.
Use your answer sheet to record your answers. You have a total of **4 prescriptions** in this station.

Station Reference: CPS – Compendium of Pharmaceuticals and Specialties

You have 7 minutes to complete this station

Written Rx 1

Rx 1
Patient Name: Reena Ming
Address:

                                                Correct date

Zestril
20 mg once daily for 4 months
Mitte: 120 tabs

T. Singh
_____ Assume signature is correct
T. Singh M.D.

Written Rx 2

Rx 2
Patient Name: Cameron Byron
Address: 3455 Sea Drive

                                                                         Correct date

Mevacor
40 mg once a day x 4 months

F. Ryan
_____ Assume signature is correct
F. Ryan M.D.

Written Rx 3

Rx 3
Patient Name: Bethany Joe
Address: 22 Heron Road

                                                                         Correct date

Niacin SR
1 g divided bid x 12 weeks

P. Wong
_____ Assume signature is correct
P. Wong M.D.

Written Rx 4

Rx 4
Patient Name: Vivian and Monica John
Address: 45 Marmot Drive

                                                          Correct date

Vibramycin
100 mg po bid on 1st day then 100 mg once daily for 5 days

T. Jacky
_____ Assume signature is correct
T. Jacky M.D.

Answer Sheet: New Prescriptions Check

Rx 1	Is this prescription ready to be processed and filled? Yes No What would you correct or add?
Rx 2	Is this prescription ready to be processed and filled? Yes No What would you correct or add?
Rx 3	Is this prescription ready to be processed and filled? Yes No What would you correct or add?
Rx 4	Is this prescription ready to be processed and filled? Yes No What would you correct or add?

Answer Key #24

Rx 1	Is this prescription ready to be processed and filled? No What would you correct or add? Missing patient's address.
Rx 2	Is this prescription ready to be processed and filled? Yes What would you correct or add? Add: take with evening meal.
Rx 3	Is this prescription ready to be processed and filled? Yes What would you correct or add? Add: Take with meals to reduce GI side effects. Swallow tablet whole. Avoid hot drinks, shot showers, spicy foods and alcohol for 1-2 hours after a dose.
Rx 4	Is this prescription ready to be processed and filled? No What would you correct or add? Two patients on the same prescription order. Add: Iron supplements and antacids reduce the absorption of Vibramycin (doxycycline)

Non Interactive Case #25: New Prescriptions Check

Candidate instructions:

Identify any mistakes, omissions or concerns on each new prescription. Some prescriptions have more than one problem. Omission of practitioner ID is not to be considered a mistake.
Use your answer sheet to record your answers. You have a total of **4 prescriptions** in this station.

Station Reference: CPS – Compendium of Pharmaceuticals and Specialties

You have 7 minutes to complete this station

Written Rx 1

Rx 1
Patient Name: Veronica George
Address: 23th North Road

                                              Correct date

Accolate
20 mg po bid x 3 months

T. Kumar
_____ Assume signature is correct
T. Kumar M.D.

Written Rx 2

```
Rx 2
Patient Name: Jeremy and Jessica Moon
Address: 345A Street


                                              Correct date



      Zenhale pMDI 100/5
      2 sprays bid x 3 months for asthma



          N. Art
     _____   Assume signature is correct
          N. Art M.D.
```

Written Rx 3

```
Rx 3
Patient Name: Minna Kim
Address: 55 Grand Road



                                              Correct date


      Losec
      20 mg qid x 15 days



          B. Xavier
     _____   Assume signature is correct
          B. Xavier M.D.
```

Written Rx 4

> Rx 4
> Patient Name: Ray Brown
> Address: 34A Spring Road
>
> Correct date
>
> Sustiva
> 600 mg once a day for 12 weeks for hepatitis B
>
> *N. Smith*
> _____ Assume signature is correct
> N. Smith M.D.

Answer Sheet: New Prescriptions Check

Rx 1	Is this prescription ready to be processed and filled? Yes No What would you correct or add?
Rx 2	Is this prescription ready to be processed and filled? Yes No What would you correct or add?
Rx 3	Is this prescription ready to be processed and filled? Yes No What would you correct or add?
Rx 4	Is this prescription ready to be processed and filled? Yes No What would you correct or add?

Answer Key #25

Rx 1	Is this prescription ready to be processed and filled? Yes What would you correct or add? Add: Take at least 1 hour before or 2 hours after meals.
Rx 2	Is this prescription ready to be processed and filled? No What would you correct or add? Two patients per order. Add: Use in the morning and evening. Prime before use with 4 test sprays. Shake well before each spray. Prime again if the inhaler is not use for 5 days. Rinse mouth following inhalation.
Rx 3	Is this prescription ready to be processed and filled? No What would you correct or add? Wrong dosing Add: ½ hour before meals
Rx 4	Is this prescription ready to be processed and filled? No What would you correct or add? Wrong drug Sustiva (Efavirenz) is used for the treatment of HIV infection.

Non Interactive Case #26: New Prescriptions Check

Candidate instructions:

Identify any mistakes, omissions or concerns on each new prescription. Some prescriptions have more than one problem. Omission of practitioner ID is not to be considered a mistake.
Use your answer sheet to record your answers. You have a total of **5 prescriptions** in this station.

Station Reference: CPS – Compendium of Pharmaceuticals and Specialties

You have 7 minutes to complete this station

Written Rx 1

Rx 1
Patient Name: Adam Hasher
Address: 55 Edmonton Avenue

Correct date

Retrovir
300 mg po for 12 months

_____ Assume signature is correct
T. June M.D.

Written Rx 2

```
Rx 2
Patient Name: Amanda Lee
Address: 222 Secondary Street

                                              Correct date


     Lumigan
     2 drop in each eye once daily for 2 weeks


        N. Matt
     _____  Assume signature is correct
        N. Matt M.D.
```

Written Rx 3

```
Rx 3
Patient Name: Nancy Peter
Address: 34 Pearl Road

                                              Correct date


     Methotrexate
     7.5 mg q12h x 6weeks for psoriasis


        P. Ali
     _____  Assume signature is correct
        P. Ali M.D.
```

Written Rx 4

```
Rx 4
Patient Name: James Troy
Address: 988 First Avenue

                                        Correct date


        Trosec
        20 mg bid x 3 months for urinary incontinence



            P. Malik
        _____    Assume signature is correct
            P. Malik M.D.
```

Written Rx 5

```
Rx 5
Patient Name: Arthur Brian
Address: 223 Second Street

                                        Correct date


        Levitra
        10 mg po 30 min before sexual activity
        Mitte: 50 tablets



            T. Park
        _____    Assume signature is correct
            T. Park M.D.
```

Answer Sheet: New Prescriptions Check

Rx 1	Is this prescription ready to be processed and filled? Yes No What would you correct or add?
Rx 2	Is this prescription ready to be processed and filled? Yes No What would you correct or add?
Rx 3	Is this prescription ready to be processed and filled? Yes No What would you correct or add?
Rx 4	Is this prescription ready to be processed and filled? Yes No What would you correct or add?
Rx 5	Is this prescription ready to be processed and filled? Yes No What would you correct or add?

Answer Key #26

Rx 1	Is this prescription ready to be processed and filled? 　　　　　　No What would you correct or add? Uncompleted dosing. Missing physician's signature
Rx 2	Is this prescription ready to be processed and filled? 　　　　　　No What would you correct or add? Missing drug strength. Lumigan is available in 0.01% or 0.03% Add: Apply in the evening.
Rx 3	Is this prescription ready to be processed and filled? 　　　　　　No What would you correct or add? Wrong dosing. 7.5 mg once a week. Add: Take folic acid supplement.
Rx 4	Is this prescription ready to be processed and filled? 　　　　　　Yes What would you correct or add? Take on empty stomach.
Rx 5	Is this prescription ready to be processed and filled? 　　　　　　Yes What would you correct or add? Add: Absorption is delayed after a meal with high fat.

Non Interactive Case #27: New Prescriptions Check

Candidate instructions:

Identify any mistakes, omissions or concerns on each new prescription. Some prescriptions have more than one problem. Omission of practitioner ID is not to be considered a mistake.
Use your answer sheet to record your answers. You have a total of **5 prescriptions** in this station.

Station Reference: CPS – Compendium of Pharmaceuticals and Specialties

You have 7 minutes to complete this station

Written Rx 1

Rx 1
Patient Name: Veronica Nasser
Address: 3th Street

Correct date

Flagyl
500 mg po q12h x 7 days
Mitte: 14 tablets

T. Moon
_____   Assume signature is correct
T. Moon M.D.

Written Rx 2

```
Rx 2
Patient Name: Pat Roger
Address: 21 Seaview Street

                                            Correct date


        Cuprimine
        500 mg once a day for rheumatoid arthritis
        Mitte: 90 tablets



            N. Cameron
    _____    Assume signature is correct
        N. Cameron M.D.
```

Written Rx 3

```
Rx 3
Patient Name: Kimberly Brent
Address: 77 Ottawa Road




        Humira
        40 mg po every other week for 12 weeks


            Y.. Chen
    _____    Assume signature is correct
        Y. Chen M.D.
```

Written Rx 4

Rx 4
Patient Name: Jacob Mason
Address: 77 Winter Drive

Correct date

Spiriva DPI
18 mg inhaled once daily for COPD
Mitte: 90 capsules

N. Phillips
_____ Assume signature is correct
N. Phillips M.D.

Written Rx 5

Rx 5
Patient Name: Dakota Zimmer
Address: 33 Horseshoe Road

Plavix
75 mg once daily x 6 months

P. Rogers
_____ Assume signature is correct
P. Rogers M.D.

Answer Sheet: New Prescriptions Check

Rx 1	Is this prescription ready to be processed and filled? Yes　　　　　　　　No What would you correct or add?
Rx 2	Is this prescription ready to be processed and filled'? Yes　　　　　　　　No What would you correct or add?
Rx 3	Is this prescription ready to be processed and filled? Yes　　　　　　　　No What would you correct or add?
Rx 4	Is this prescription ready to be processed and filled? Yes　　　　　　　　No What would you correct or add?
Rx 5	Is this prescription ready to be processed and filled? Yes　　　　　　　　No What would you correct or add?

Answer Key #27

Rx 1	Is this prescription ready to be processed and filled? Yes What would you correct or add? Add: Avoid alcohol until 48 hours after the last dose to prevent disulfiram-like reaction Disulfiram, chloramphenicol, furazolidone, metronidazole, and quinacrine are reported to produce a disulfiram-like reaction or alcohol intolerance due to the inhibition of hepatic aldehyde dehydrogenase; symptoms include headaches, palpitations and flushing.
Rx 2	Is this prescription ready to be processed and filled? Yes What would you correct or add? Add: Take on empty stomach
Rx 3	Is this prescription ready to be processed and filled? No What would you correct or add? Wrong administration route; sc instead of po. 40 mg/0.8 ml injection. Missing date.
Rx 4	Is this prescription ready to be processed and filled? No What would you correct or add? Wrong dosing/drug strength. It should be 18 ug tiotropium (1 capsule). Administer by inhalation using the HandiHaler device.
Rx 5	Is this prescription ready to be processed and filled? No What would you correct or add? Missing date

Made in the USA
Middletown, DE
15 April 2019